AFTER WORK

The
Search
for an
Optimal
Leisure
Lifestyle

*Robert A.
Stebbins*

Detselig Enterprises Ltd.

Calgary, Alberta, Canada

After Work

© 1998 Robert A. Stebbins

Canadian Cataloguing in Publication Data

Stebbins, Robert A., 1938-
  After work

Includes bibliographical references and index.
ISBN 1-55059-157-6

1. Leisure. I. Title
GV14.45.S73 1998   790.01   C97-910998-1

Detselig Enterprises Ltd.
210-1220 Kensington Rd. N.W.
Calgary, Alberta T2N 3P5

Detselig Enterprises Ltd. appreciates the financial support for our 1998 publishing program, provided by Canadian Heritage and the Alberta Foundation for the Arts, a beneficiary of the Lottery Fund of the Government of Alberta.

Printed in Canada
ISBN 1-55059-157-6
SAN 115-0324

Cover design by Dean Macdonald

To David and Barbara Todd

Table of Contents

Acknowledgments

I wish to thank Cynthia Janzen for her careful work on several aspects of the Practical Bibliography and the Social Sciences and Humanities Research Council of Canada for the small research grant that made it possible to pay her for her efforts. I am also grateful to my wife, Karin Stebbins, for typing that bibliography. Finally, I deeply appreciate the efforts of Linda Berry, whose copyediting has greatly enhanced this book.

Introduction

I wrote *After Work* with two audiences in mind. One is those self-directed learners searching for an optimal leisure lifestyle, which I conceive as the pursuit, during free time, of a substantial, absorbing leisure activity. The other consists of leisure practitioners and students in leisure studies and continuing education who would like to help people realize their free-time goals. The scientific basis for this book lies in the field of serious leisure research, a relatively new branch of the leisure sciences. Some of the people seeking an optimal leisure lifestyle today have had their jobs made redundant, some have retired (whether at, before or after age 65) and some, though still fully employed, are bored with their present leisure lifestyle. Those who succeed in their search will discover and embrace one of three types of serious leisure: the steady pursuit of an amateur, hobbyist or career volunteer activity that captivates them with its challenges and complexity.

Several writers, among them Jeremy Rifkin, Ann Howard, and Stanley Aronowitz and William DiFazio, have observed that the number of people with substantial free time on their hands is growing dramatically, paralleling the rapid spread of electronic technology and the sharp reduction in job opportunities that nearly always follows. One consequence is that, to find the same identity, respect and focus they once knew in their work, more and more people will be forced to find a free-time activity with the same substance. *After Work* takes us down the road to the Leisure Age, exploring along the way the complex world of serious leisure as well as practical questions of how to get started in the amateur, hobbyist or volunteer activities that pique our interest.

My interest in serious leisure dates to 1974 when I began my theoretical work on this concept. Since then I have conducted practical studies of 11 serious leisure activities: amateurs in baseball, Canadian football, archaeology, astronomy, theater, classical music, entertainment magic and stand-up comedy; hobbyists in barbershop singing and cultural tourism; and volunteers in the French communities of Calgary and Edmonton. I continue to work on the theory, expanding the perspective as well as linking it with areas of similar interest, mainly tourism, well-being, philosophy, volunteering and continuing education. Since I refer to these studies without citation, if you would like to know more about them, search the entries under my name in "Works Cited." Because they were field studies and because I wrote them as much for the people I observed and interviewed as for my professional colleagues, the books and articles listed are not technically difficult. Many others have also contributed to our knowledge about these activities; they *are* properly cited in the text and referenced.

Although this book is about serious leisure and the benefits it offers all of us, I open it with an examination of the larger social and economic backdrop for contemporary leisure, that of revolutionary electronic technology, a force now engulfing everyone. Here, after discussing the essential characteristics of serious leisure, I describe its three principal types and then explore the satisfaction they can bring, which is never free of costs. I then turn to the practical matter of getting started in one or two of the more than 300 serious leisure activities. Many of you will find the Practical Bibliography of Serious Leisure, which contains short lists of introductory books on most of these activities, of further help.

An examination of social and personal identity, leisure lifestyle and leisure marginality follows. In the final chapter I explore how we can make the transition from the Industrial Age and the need-to-work life to the Leisure Age and a life of serious leisure, a difficult process for many. The day is approaching when most people can enjoy an optimal leisure lifestyle, even if many must first clear certain critical social, personal and economic hurdles before they can partake of it.

Chapter 1

Leisure in the Information Age

Today, as always, people are searching for answers, and it may be that if they can see leisure not as a problem but, rather, as an *opportunity* for enriching their lives, they may become less apathetic about the prospect of being defeated by an empty hour.

I have assumed that most of us measure *opportunity* in terms of what *we* want from life, and that given time free from the things we must do to stay alive, we can have a personally satisfying and full existence through *recreative* living. (Charles K. Brightbill, *Man and Leisure*)

"After work" – for many people these two words have an alluring ring, implying the happy time in life when we may do what we want to do, to be sure, always limited by our mental, physical, financial and situational resources. These limits aside, for most people, the list of all their possible after-work activities is remarkably long and, were they entirely familiar with it, they would have trouble deciding which held the greatest appeal for them. Still, it is not so bad to have to choose among agreeable options; whatever you choose, it will be welcome, one of the most important qualities of the activities people engage in after work.

In this book, after work refers to both much more and much less than the hours and days of our paid employment. First, if the hours after work are to be agreeable, then they cannot include such disagreeable tasks of everyday life as washing the dishes, shoveling the sidewalk and going to the dentist. Though done during non-work time, these are classified by most people as something quite other than after-work activities. Still, if someone finds pleasure in shoveling a sidewalk, then that lucky person can proclaim this an after work activity and pray for the next snowstorm.

In other words, the time after work is free time. This time, however, refers to free time available at all stages of life. For instance, there are people whose time after work is their retirement or their unemployment. Unfortunately, some of these non-workers have been subjected to unwanted free time, because they have been forced to retire early or, in the case of unemployment, have been forced to leave work temporarily.

Today in the industrialized world there is more time after work than ever. Still, it was true for awhile in the United States, as Juliet Schor pointed out in 1991 in *The Overworked American*, that many people were so eager to make money that they took a second job or worked overtime, striving to save money through do-it-yourself projects. After meeting the obligations they had set for themselves, these drudges found themselves with next to no free time. By 1995, however, Christine Howe could write that this attitude was changing; now more and more American workers were emphasizing "reasoned wellness" while backing off from the greed and narcissism of earlier years.[1] They were also beginning to treat family time as having the same importance as work and obligated time. In a similar vein, Samuel described the tendency observed by Schor as a "temporary development" in the United States that stands out against the world-wide trend toward increased free time.[2]

Overall, the after-work time of many people has started to grow both in amount and significance. Moreover, this trend continues despite the tendency for managers to wring extra hours of service from their employees.[3] My observations suggest that these employees, drowned in work as they are, cannot surface long enough to notice that many others are thirsting for the work they have in excess. Yet, the size of this group of reluctantly overworked employees is shrinking as more of their positions are lost to electronic technology.

Bernard Lefkowitz foresaw this trend – the intentional, substantial reduction of life's work and non-work obligations – in his book, *Breaktime*. His interviews, conducted during the late 1970s, suggested that a small but growing number of Americans were expanding their leisure involvements by voluntarily accepting unemployment, partial employment or early retirement. Two years later Daniel Yankelovich confirmed these impressions in a survey reported in *New Rules*. Today, the evidence supports the idea that the work ethic of old is waning in intensity, even in North America, the home of the largest number of its supporters by far.

But paralleling the tendency to voluntarily cut back on work time is a much stronger force: the technologically-driven, involuntary reduction of paid work. In *The End of Work*, Jeremy Rifkin describes the current decline in the size of the global labor pool and the traditional market economy and how both forces are now pushing ever larger numbers of people toward greater free time at an alarming rate, whatever their interest in reducing their level of work. As the 21st century approaches, many employable people are finding that job opportunities have shrunk, sometimes to nothing at all. Behind these unsettling trends lie the powerful forces of what Rifkin calls the "Third Industrial Revolution": the far-reaching effects of electronic technology such as computers, robotics, telecommunications and similar devices.

The Information Age has dawned. In it, Rifkin observes, these technologies will continue well into the 21st century, replacing workers in every sector of the economy, including manufacturing, transportation, agriculture, government and the retail and financial services. New jobs will be created in significant numbers only in the knowledge sector, in science, computing, consulting, education and the technical and professional services directly related to the new technology. Rifkin says this sector will compose no more than 20% of the work force. Jobs lost in the other sectors will be gone forever, offset very little by the small number of jobs generated in the knowledge sector. Occupational retraining is no solution, for the people eligible for it generally lack the necessary education on which to build the skills and information they would need to work in the knowledge sector. In short, regardless of the modern person's attitude toward life after work, we are now destined to have much more of it than ever before. Two other books by Stanley Aronowitz and William DiFazio (*The Jobless Future*) and Ann Howard (*The Changing Nature of Work*) indicate that Rifkin is not alone in observing these trends.[4]

What will we do with our newfound free time? These writers have failed to address this question, other than making two broad observations, one tantalizing, the other frightening. They predict that the Information Age will offer greatly expanded opportunities for leisure, personal development and time far in excess of our capacity to use constructively. From the standpoint of someone trying to adapt to a world of momentous change, these observers sketch a picture about life after work in the Information Age that is much too hazy for comfort.[5]

The task I have set for myself in this book is to complete this picture, to sharpen its focus and to explore in detail the activities that people can pursue in their time after work. I describe opportunities for personal development available in "serious leisure," showing how to use whatever free time is available to achieve an optimal leisure lifestyle. Bear in mind as we go along that serious leisure knows no demographic boundaries; it is as appropriate for men as for women, for adolescents as for retirees, for the fully employed as for the permanently unemployed. Gail Sheehy observes in *New Passages* that at least half the baby boomers can expect to live healthy, active lives well into their 80s and 90s. They, too, can participate in a number of serious leisure activities. Nevertheless, some of the activities discussed in the next three chapters will appeal chiefly to males or females or to certain age groups.

Leisure as a Personal and Social Good

The quotation from Charles Brightbill, with which I introduced this chapter, indicates that leisure is activity we intentionally choose because it brings us pleasure or, in more profound leisure, satisfaction. Even if the activity is sedentary, such as taking a nap or watching passersby, it is leisure if the napper or the watcher has chosen it. This is why free time, or the time after work, is usually not the same as leisure. Most people pass at least a few minutes each day where they do nothing, as in daydreaming, watching the world go by or twiddling their thumbs. During these moments they are either bored or resting, both being aimless states. This use of free time is most common among the unemployed, and the research of Sue Glyptis and Tess Kay, among others, shows that the time the unemployed spend waiting for work is often filled with boredom.[6] These examples portray free time, then, rather than leisure as I have defined it.

Leisure's qualities of choice and pleasure or satisfaction go hand in hand with a third quality: initiative. It is up to us to seek our own leisure, whatever that may be. Leisure will not come to us; rather we must go to it, choosing what we can do and then pursuing it. So far as leisure is concerned, people are responsible for their own happiness or lack of it. Although there are limits on leisure choice, no one is completely without choices no matter how small their number.

Today, most people see leisure as a good thing, an important social and personal value. True, leisure was not always held in such high esteem, particularly among people influenced by the Protestant ethic, who once wrote it off as mere recreation. In their view, the time after work was to be spent resting up for life's most important activity – work – which they saw as the only sure road to salvation in the next life. Although this understanding of leisure is not entirely passé today, it is less common than before.

Witold Rybczynski tells of leisure's contemporary meaning in his book *Waiting for the Weekend*. In North America, and perhaps some other parts of the world, people often celebrate the start of the weekend by quipping "thank God it's Friday" or simply "TGIF." The Swiss sociologist Christian Lalive D'Epinay holds that, especially in Europe, but even in North America to some extent, the distinction between work and leisure is now dissolving.[7] Instead of identifying themselves by their occupation and place of work, people increasingly identify themselves by their most meaningful form of leisure, or by a combination of the two. Although Lalive D'Epinay didn't address this question, it is clear that if leisure is to fill this role it must somehow generate significant satisfaction. If it is only weakly satisfying, it risks being no more distinctive than the jobs many people hold. Leisure is not likely to become an identity peg under these conditions.

Even though they often agree that leisure is a good thing, many people have little or no idea how to find the leisure leading to the greatest personal satisfaction and an optimal leisure lifestyle. E.M. Forster reflects on the problem in *A Passage to India*:

> Most of life is so dull that there is nothing to be said about it, and the books and talk that would describe it as interesting are obligated to exaggerate, in the hope of justifying their own existence. Inside its cocoon of work or social obligation, the human spirit slumbers for the most part, registering the

distinction between pleasure and pain, but not nearly so alert as we pretend.

Forster is saying that, although some of this is leisure – it is not boredom – it is nonetheless rather dull, humdrum leisure.

Yet, some people do manage to find an exciting, absorbing leisure activity. Consider the following three contrasting leisure lifestyles:

Mark – Regenerative Leisure

Mark is a data analyst at Ajax Engineering. He puts in long hours because, as a salaried employee, he is expected to fulfill his duties no matter how long it takes. After work, particularly on weekends, he economizes by completing the occasional do-it-yourself project around the house. Life for Mark is filled mostly with obligations, with very little time for play. He has no hobbies. Rather, what little leisure he has comes from watching television. For Mark television is recreational, a way of regenerating himself for the obligations of the next day. His leisure offers him few benefits apart from this.

Nancy – Diverse Casual Leisure

Nancy's job as a department manager for a large wholesale firm seldom requires her to work overtime. Since she lives alone in an apartment, the number of domestic chores is small. Consequently, during her evenings and weekends, she is largely free to pursue the leisure of her choice. Here Nancy likes variety, but nothing too demanding. Sometimes she watches television at home alone, but preferring to be with friends, she spends most of her leisure hours with them, dining out, attending films, going dancing, walking in city parks and passing hours in coffee houses and jazz clubs listening to music and talking. After a couple of hours, any one of these activities becomes boring, forcing Nancy to find something else to do. She enjoys her leisure lifestyle because of the variety it offers.

Tom and Marge – Serious Leisure

Tom and Marge are married and own their own house. He is a building contractor, she teaches elementary school. Although they are homeowners, neither cares much for routine domestic chores. Rather than do these things themselves, they either ignore them or hire someone to do them. Since both must occasionally work long hours at their jobs, they avoid activities that would take time away from their leisure passion: barbershop singing. Each belongs to a chorus and a quartet, but not the same ones, since mixed groups are rare in this art. Performing, practicing and rehearsing consume a great deal of after-work time each week. Marge also serves as the publicity coordinator for her chorus, which is not a hobby, but a volunteer role. Tom and Marge's leisure lifestyle is powerfully attractive because they find it enriching and rewarding in terms of personal growth.

In principle, then, leisure is a good thing. But in everyday life people often have trouble finding leisure activities capable of generating the sort of deep satisfaction that Tom and Marge have found, activities that can serve as the basis for an optimal leisure lifestyle.

Finding the Right Leisure

Mark, Nancy, Tom and Marge have all found a kind of leisure in their after-work activities. If questioned on it, each would likely say their leisure lifestyle was good, even though in-depth interviews would show that Tom and Marge gain much more from theirs than Nancy, who still gains much more than Mark. This unequal return on free time raises at least two important questions: Are Mark and Nancy *aware* that more satisfying leisure is available (again within their mental, physical, financial and situational constraints)? There are over 300 serious leisure activities to consider. Second, if and when they become aware of the existence of more satisfying leisure, *should* they seek it?

Turning to the first question, John Neulinger points out in *To Leisure* that some people suffer from a "leisure lack." When they have too little leisure, they are motivated to fill this void in their lives. Both Mark and Nancy have their leisure activities. What they lack is an awareness of the many alternatives, especially the ones that are highly satisfying. One might be tempted to say that this is a case where ignorance is bliss and let the matter rest at that. But Forster's observation about the dullness of much of life compels us to do something. A major goal in leisure studies is to identify, examine and publicize the vast range of leisure alternatives, to help people find and pursue those activities they will find most satisfying.

As for the second question, no one should be telling other people what leisure to pursue. A main part of the appeal of leisure is the freedom to choose it. Nevertheless, leisure science can draw up an annotated list of leisure activities, highlighting and recommending those that can generate high levels of satisfaction. After looking over the list, people could select those activities within their limits with the greatest appeal. Obviously, most people do not need leisure science to help them find casual leisure, Mark's and Nancy's leisure. It is common leisure, familiar to everyone who takes part in the everyday life of the local community. But leisure science can help people find the type of leisure pursued by Tom and Marge, serious leisure. Serious leisure is much less common than its casual cousin and more often hidden from public view in the activities of individuals and small groups. This is the high-reward leisure that leisure science has only recently begun to identify and explore. My argument is that people searching for an optimal leisure lifestyle will most likely find it in the sphere of serious leisure.

Serious Leisure

Serious leisure stands in contrast to "casual" or "unserious" leisure, which poses fewer challenges, is much simpler in structure and rarely requires a steady commitment to perform it well. Although an oversimplification, casual leisure can be described as all leisure falling outside the three basic types of serious leisure. There is a bewildering array of casual forms, among them strolling in the park, observing a fireworks display, going on a picnic and taking an afternoon nap.[8]

Amateurs are found in art, science, sport and entertainment, where they are linked with their professional counterparts. The two can be distinguished by the fact that professionals make a living at it. Furthermore, professionals work full-time at the activity, whereas amateurs pursue it part-time.[9] Part-time professionals in art and entertainment complicate this picture; although they work part-time, their work is judged by other professionals and by amateurs as being of professional quality. As the Third Industrial Revolution unfolds, part-time professionals are likely to become more common not only in art and entertainment, but also in science and possibly even in sport.

Hobbyists lack this professional alter ego, even though they sometimes have commercial equivalents and often have small publics who take an interest in what they do. Leisure science classifies the scores of hobbyists into five categories: collectors; makers and tinkers; activity participants; competitors in sports, games and contests; and enthusiasts in the liberal arts fields. Some hobbies evolve into professions, transforming the hobbyists into amateurs along the way. This transition has been made at different points in history by all the amateur-professional fields in art, science, sport and entertainment. The commercial equivalents of hobbies, such as making and selling furniture or trout flies, are more accurately viewed as businesses than professions.

No one knows how many hobbies there are. Collectors alone abound in every imaginable field, some well known, such as those who collect stamps or coins; some more obscure, such as those who collect juke boxes or lapel pins. Making and tinkering is a somewhat more limited hobby. Besides making (or building) such items as flies and furniture, these hobbyists tinker with or repair cars or various gadgets around the house, for example. Activity participants find their leisure in a range of non-competitive, rule-based pursuits, including fishing, bird-watching and barbershop singing. By contrast, competitors in games, sports and contests thrive on competition. They go in for field hockey, long-distance running or competitive swimming, among others, activities where no professional counterparts exist. Liberal arts hobbyists love the systematic acquisition of knowledge for its own sake. Many of them read voraciously in art, sport, cuisine, language, culture, history, science, philosophy, politics or literature. Some of them expand their knowledge still further through cultural travel.[10]

Volunteers – the third basic type – engage in volunteering, described by Jon Van Til in *Mapping the Third Sector* (p. 6) as:

> a helping action of an individual that is valued by him or her and yet is not aimed directly at material gain or mandated or coerced by others. Thus, in the broadest sense, *volunteering*

is an uncoerced helping activity that is engaged in not primarily for financial gain and not by coercion or mandate. It is thereby different in definition from work, slavery, or conscription.

Volunteering as serious leisure is different from volunteering as casual leisure. In serious leisure volunteering, people find a (non-work) career in acquiring special skills, knowledge or training and, at times, two or three of these. In this regard, David Ross found in his Canadian survey that the overwhelming majority of volunteers define these acquisitions as important and look on volunteer work as a satisfying and convenient way of using them.[11] He grouped the acquired skills and knowledge according to whether they were interpersonal, communications, fund-raising, technical and office, or organizational and managerial. These skills are substantial enough to create a career of acquiring them and applying them. They contrast with giving blood, distributing flyers or taking tickets at performances of the local community theater, all instances of casual volunteering too simple and transitory to qualify as career volunteering. These last require no significant development of skill or knowledge.

Although career volunteering is only part of the vast domain of volunteering, it nonetheless covers considerable ground. Statistics Canada lists seven types of organizations within which career volunteers provide different services: health (physical and non-physical health care for all ages), educational (service inside and outside the formal school system), social/welfare (child care, family counselling, correctional services), leisure (service in athletic and non-athletic associations), religious (service in religious organizations), civic/community action (advocacy, service in professional and labor organizations) and political (service in political organizations).[12] Although much of career volunteering is connected with organizations, the scope of this leisure is even broader, including the kinds of help individuals devote to social movements or to family and neighbors. Still, the definition of serious leisure restricts attention to volunteering in which we can find a career, in which we offer more or less continuous, substantial help, rather than a one-time donation of money, organs or services.

Serious leisure is further defined by distinctive qualities found among amateurs, hobbyists and career volunteers alike.

One of these qualities is *perseverance*. For example, Gary Fine tells of the dangers faced by the collectors of wild mushrooms who eat their harvest, while George Floro describes the embarrassment endured by those who volunteer in certain fields. I found stage fright to be a common problem for amateurs in sport and theater.[13] Yet to some extent, positive feelings about the activity come from sticking with it through thick and thin, from conquering adversity.

Another quality distinguishing all three types of serious leisure is the opportunity to follow a *career* in the endeavor shaped by its own special chance events, turning points, stages of achievement and involvement. From a sociological perspective, careers are not limited to the world of work; they can also be pursued in other complicated roles, including the serious leisure roles. Moreover, most, if not all, of these careers owe their existence to a third quality: serious leisure participants make a significant personal *effort* based on specially acquired *knowledge*, *training* or *skill* and at times, all three. Thus, the careers of serious leisure participants consist of their efforts to achieve a high level of achievement, knowledge or experience.

Serious leisure is further distinguished by a number of *durable benefits*, the tangible, beneficial outcomes we get out of such activity. They are self-fulfillment, cherished experiences, self-expression, renewed energy and interest in life, feelings of accomplishment, enhanced self-esteem, meeting people and making friends, belonging to groups and lasting physical products (e.g., a painting, scientific paper, piece of furniture). A further benefit – pure fun – is by far the least lasting benefit in this list. Realizing such benefits is a powerful goal in serious leisure.

The fifth quality – participants in serious leisure tend to *identify* strongly with their chosen pursuits – springs from the other distinctive qualities. In contrast, casual leisure is too fleeting, mundane and commonplace to become the basis for a distinctive identity for most people. I should imagine this was the quality Cicero had in mind when he coined his famous slogan: *otium cum dignitate*, which translates as "leisure with dignity."

Finally, serious leisure is distinguished by the *unique character or spirit* that emerges in reference to each expression of it. A central component of this spirit is the special social world which takes shape when enthusiasts pursue substantial shared interests over many years. According to David Unruh, every social world has its characteristic groups, events, routines, practices and organizations. It is held together by semiformal, or mediated, communication. In other words, social worlds are neither heavily bureaucratic nor substantially organized through personal interaction. Rather, communication is through newsletters, posted notices, telephone messages, mass mailings, radio and television announcements and similar means.[14]

The social world is a formless entity, but still important in the impersonal, segmented life of the modern urban community, where formal work organizations are now becoming increasingly marginal in everyday affairs. Part of this importance comes from the freedom people have to enter it (given the right qualifications) and leave it. Part comes from their voluntary identification with the social world and its central activities – e.g., gun collecting, amateur chamber music, volunteer fire fighting. Moreover, because they are so diffuse, it is common for people to be only partly involved in the full range of activities the social world has to offer. After all, a social world may be local, regional, multi-regional, national, even international. In my book *The Barbershop Singer,* I describe the organization of male and female barbershop singing, a hobby spanning all five levels. Finally, people in complex societies are commonly members of several social worlds, only some of which have to do with leisure.

Unruh notes that every social world has different types of members, whom he refers to as strangers, tourists, regulars and insiders. Strangers are intermediaries who participate little in the leisure activity itself, but who do something important to make it possible, for example, by managing municipal parks (in amateur baseball), minting coins (in hobbyist coin collecting) and organizing the work of teachers' aides (in career volunteering). Tourists are temporary participants in a social world; they come for profit, advantage or entertainment. Most amateur and hobbyist activities have publics which, for our purposes, can be called tourists. The clients of many volunteers can be similarly classified. The regulars routinely participate in their social world; in serious leisure, they are the amateurs, hobbyists and volunteers. The insiders are those among them who show exceptional devotion to maintaining and advancing the social world they share.[15]

Missing from Unruh's idea of the social world, yet vitally important for the study of serious leisure, is the idea that it is also a rich subculture. In other words, there is in each social world a set of special norms, values, beliefs, styles, moral principles, performance standards and shared representations. These elements help explain the social ranking that occurs in every social world; for example, how else than by such criteria as norms, values and performance standards can we explain Unruh's observation about the differences in prestige and motivation distinguishing insiders from regulars?

Serious Leisure as a Substitute for Work

The social world is not only a concept well in tune with work and leisure routines, it is also desired by many, both for today and for the years to come. If people cannot belong to a work organization or can only belong as an outside consultant or part-time employee, where can they connect themselves with the community, whether local, regional, national or international? Increasingly, the only available communal connections for most people will come through their after-work activities. Because they tend to be private, family activities cannot usually provide such connections. But one of the principal attractions of an amateur, hobbyist or volunteer activity is the sense of being part of its bustling, fascinating, all-encompassing social world. For many enthusiasts this involvement is as exciting as the activity itself and, in volunteer work, often indistinguishable from it.

For people who have too little work or no work at all, the routines of serious leisure activities can be appealing. Many amateur activities require regular practice and rehearsal sessions. Volunteers are often asked to serve at regular times. People who miss the routine of the full-time job can often find an equivalent at least as satisfying in one of more serious leisure pursuits.

In the next four chapters I will explore the various social worlds associated with the three types of serious leisure and show the enormous range of possibilities they hold for an optimal leisure lifestyle. This includes an examination of the kinds of leisure careers available. In Chapter 6 I provide descriptive lists of the activities found in each type of serious leisure, giving a complete list for the amateur activities and lengthy selected lists for the hobbies and volunteer involvements. The activities of the second and third types are too numerous to cover in their entirety, and some are even obscure enough to have escaped my attention.

Notes

[1]Howe, "Factors Impacting Leisure in Middle Aged Adults throughout the World."

[2]Samuel, "The Future of Leisure Time," p. 48.

[3]This practice of mandatory overtime for existing employees is said to cost the employer significantly less than hiring additional employees. For instance, management economizes by avoiding the costs of fringe benefits for new personnel.

[4]These authors are by no means the first analysts to note these trends. For example, Clive Jenkins and Barrie Sherman discussed them from a British standpoint in 1979 in *The Collapse of Work*. Three years later in *Sleepers, Wake! Technology and the Future of Work*, Barry Jones described the same processes at work in Australia. Nevertheless, Rifkin was able to observe in 1995 (p. 6) that enormous corporate spending during the 1980s on electronic technology began to pay off only in the early 1990s through increased productivity, reduced labor costs and greater profits. The cost of labor is being reduced chiefly by shrinking the work force.

[5]See, for example, Jenkins and Sherman's *The Leisure Shock* and Sherman's *Working at Leisure*. Rifkin comes closer than the others to completing the story when he examines the role of volunteers and community service in the closing chapters of his book.

[6]Sue Glyptis, *Leisure and Unemployment*; Tess Kay, "Active Unemployment."

[7]Lalive D'Epinay, "Beyond the Antinomy."

[8]For a more thorough discussion of this form of leisure, see Stebbins, "Casual Leisure: A Conceptual Statement."

[9]These are common sense ways of distinguishing amateurs from professionals. In my research on these two types, the professionals are identified and defined according to theory developed in the social scientific study of professions, a substantially more exact procedure than the simplistic and not infrequently commercially-shaped common sense images of these workers (see Stebbins, *Amateurs, Professionals, and Serious Leisure*).

[10]The liberal arts hobbies are examined in greater detail in two articles I wrote titled "The Liberal Arts Hobbies" and "Cultural Tourism as Serious Leisure."

[11]David P. Ross, "Economic Dimensions of Volunteer Work in Canada," pp. 20-27.

[12]Statistics Canada, *An Overview of Volunteer Workers in Canada*.

[13]Fine, "Dying for a Laugh"; Floro, "What to Look for in a Study of the Volunteer in the Work World"; Stebbins, "Toward a Social Psychology of Stage Fright."

[14]These ideas on the social world are drawn from Unruh, "The Nature of Social Worlds" and "Characteristics and Types of Participation in Social Worlds."

[15]In the studies of amateurs and hobbyists, such people have often been analyzed as "devotees" and compared with "participants," who are the regulars in Unruh's scheme (see Stebbins, *Amateurs, professionals, and serious leisure*, p. 46). To keep the terminology simple, I will use Unruh's terms throughout.

Chapter

2

Amateurism and the Love of Leisure

As professionalization spreads from one occupation to another, what was once considered play has been evolving into modern amateurism. Modern amateurism has been evolving alongside those occupations to the point that workers are now able to make a substantial living from them and devote themselves to those occupations as vocations rather than as avocations. Although there are others, science, entertainment, sport and games, as well as the fine arts, are the major occupational areas where work was once purely play and where modern amateurism now has a parallel development.

Those who play at the activities encompassed by these occupations are being overrun in significance, if not in numbers, by professionals and amateurs. The process appears to unfold as follows. As opportunities for full-time pursuit of a skill or activity gradually appear, those people with even an average aptitude can develop it to a higher level than the part-time participant. With the availability of professional performances and products, new standards of excellence soon confront all participants, professional or not. Although the performances of professionals are impressive, no one is more impressed than the non-professionals who, through direct experience, know the activity intimately. Indeed, once they become aware of the professional standards, all they have accomplished can seem mediocre by comparison. They are thus faced with a critical choice: either they don't identify with the activity so as to remain unaffected by such unfair comparisons, or they identify with it and attempt to meet those standards.

The first choice is still common. The part-time participant then remains a player, dabbler or dilettante. Drawing on Johan Huizinga's ideas on play in *Homo Ludens*, we can say that this type of leisure lacks necessity, obligation and utility and is produced with a disinterest that sets it apart from the participants' ordinary, real lives. Play is then a type of casual leisure.

The second choice is also common and becoming more so. It drives part-time participants toward the pursuit of durable benefits and serious leisure. These benefits, however, are built on necessity, obligation, seriousness and commitment, as expressed in rehearsals and practices and schedules and organization. Most of the travelers on this road will reach amateur status, while a few will journey farther to become professionals.

The Modern Amateur

Not everyone views the rise of the modern amateur in the same favorable light. Jacques Godbout, for example, scornfully labelled this trend the "professionalization of leisure," pointing to such qualities as obligation, regimentation and systematization as evidence for his claim.[1] When I have discussed with friends my research on amateurs or my own amateur involvements, it is not unusual for them to say that such leisure "sounds alot like work."

Although amateurs describe their activities as leisure, the activities and their relations with their professional counterparts do resemble work in several ways. For instance, amateurs serve publics as professionals do and, at times, even the same ones. Amateurs are also driven by the standards of excellence set and communicated by the latter. Some university baseball teams play before crowds of fans who also attend professional games. There are situations, as in theatre, in which the local public has little opportunity to take in anything other than amateur productions, which are frequently lauded for their high quality.

Moreover, financial and organizational relationships are often established when professionals educate, train, direct, coach, advise, organize and even perform with amateurs, and when amateurs are part of their public. For example, amateurs can be found among the spectators watching a professional baseball game the week after the amateurs' game. Likewise, when a professional theatre company visits a community where an amateur theatre group exists, many of the latter will attend the performance. Similarly, amateurs play with professionals in "pro-am" bowling and in open tournaments in golf, squash and tennis. Indeed, these two types are often members of the same orchestra or theatre group. As for the sciences, amateur projects are sometimes reported in professional journals as well as in journals devoted partly or wholly to amateur work (e.g., *The Local Historian*, *Sky and Telescope*, *The Bulletin of the Amateur Entomologists' Society*).

Another work-related relationship joining amateurs and professionals centers on their career paths. Professionals with amateur counterparts typically start out as amateurs and, unless they abandon their pursuit entirely or die before they retire, they return to amateur status, often as the final stage of their career. In an age where professionals in art, science, sport and entertainment receive the lion's share of public attention while amateurs are mostly ignored, we need to be reminded from time to time that amateurism is the seedbed of professionalism in these four areas.

Both amateurs and professionals possess extensive knowledge of the theory and technique related to their field. Granted, the professionals are generally more fully trained and experienced. Yet to qualify as experts or practitioners, both must use their knowledge and technique often enough to prevent them from degenerating. Even the idea of amateur presupposes consistently active use of the knowledge and core skills of a particular field. Today's extensive free time makes this possible.[2]

Finally, amateur involvement in an activity is possible only when the training, licensing and equipment are available to those who intend to make it an avocation. Few people are likely to go through formal medical training merely to practice medicine as an amateur, whereas those without this training would be refused legal recognition. According to the definition of amateurism developed here, the practice of amateur law, nursing, medicine, primary and secondary education and the like are for the most part legal impossibilities. One never hears the people who provide these services referred to in everyday conversation as amateurs, unless by "amateur" the speaker means "quack" or "imposter." Indeed, the training for police officers and airline pilots, since it is less rigorous than training for physicians, is more available to would-be amateurs. But official authorization to assume these roles would be denied amateurs, as would the necessary equipment, such as uniforms, badges, patrol cars and commercial airplanes. Thus there can be neither amateur police officers nor amateur airline pilots unless, as the police have done on occasion, citizen patrol units are given official authorization.[3]

We can conclude that amateurs engage in part-time activities that are full-time work for other people. You cannot be an amateur butterfly catcher or matchbook collector; no full-time employment exists in those areas. Rather, these are hobbies; as such they lie outside the professional-amateur-public relations discussed here.

We can also conclude that, even for amateurs, there is nearly always a public of some kind. Perhaps they (as well as professionals) imagine a public once in awhile. Their real public may be small, mainly friends, neighbors, relatives and other amateurs in the same activity. Nonetheless, much of the time most amateurs are serving a public, not simply themselves. In fact, since they can only be carried out in groups, many pursuits are social in and of themselves. Here the public is made up in part of other participants. However, lone guitarists, piano players and other solitary participants in serious leisure are excluded from this aspect of amateur life. Viewed from this angle, they are not amateurs at all.

Whereas amateurs are not professionals, they are also neither dabblers nor novices. Dabblers are casual leisure participants with levels of technique, knowledge and active involvement in the field that barely distinguish them from the public. Every amateur-professional field seems to have a number of them, including science, in which books are published with instructions on how to amuse oneself and others with simple scientific procedures.[4]

Novices are people who may someday be amateurs, possibly even professionals. They, too, form a special part of the supporting public. They are beginners who consistently pursue the activity (thus they are more than mere dabblers), but who have yet to grow proficient and knowledgeable enough to be considered amateurs. Neither dabblers nor novices are apt to refer to themselves as practitioners in their activity. Statements like "I'm just learning to sculpt" or "I just fool around at golf" identify these people. In other words, amateurs, while recognizing their limitations, identify themselves as more seriously involved. In his autobiography, *At Home with Music*, amateur cellist Leonard Marsh argues that

> it is time to recognize that amateurs are not necessarily novices. Everybody has to start as a novice, including even composers and conductors; they do not need remain so. If they are willing to study, practise and to learn, they will build in something for good . . . Toscanini was one of the Great amateurs: he loved the music with the divine passion of the saint. I don't claim anything at these altitudes, being a very gentle and I hope, non-fanatical, amateur. But I can testify to the determination to play it well (pp. 168-169).

We can learn still more about the modern amateur by considering the Latin roots of the word "amateur;" an *amator*, is one who loves. This definition, often naively used, needs qualification. First, although it is possible that amateurs are attracted to their pursuits more than their professional colleagues (perhaps because they engage in them less often), the activity is not always pure joy for either. Amateurs get tired, bored, peeved, frustrated and discouraged just as professionals do; acquiring, maintaining and expressing skill and knowledge is certain to bring on such feelings from time to time. As an example, consider the avocational archaeologist. Excavation is arduous. Digging, hauling and sifting dirt for hours on end in an environment of burs, heat, insects and humidity (depending on the locale) requires a stamina and devotion to archaeology that will put off some novices. More than once I've heard people say they would rebel against such labor were it a job requirement.

Entertainment and the Fine Arts

The fine arts appeal to the mind and to our sense of beauty. Many artistic works also convey a powerful social or emotional message such as ethnic injustice, national treason or personal ruin. By comparison, most entertainment rests on pure humor or on pure amusement, on easily understood material not designed to absorb the intellect or prick the conscience. Nevertheless, the relationship between these two fields is complex, which explains why they are treated in the same section of this book.

Part of this relationship rests on the twin facts that both fields are arts and share many techniques. For the most part these techniques originated in the fine arts and then flowed from there to the entertainment world. Today a properly trained rock trumpeter will have received lessons in classical trumpet, giving the trumpeter a solid base for making music as an entertainer. A person planning a career in Broadway theater learns the same fundamentals as the person planning a career on the Shakespearean stage. Exceptions do exist, nevertheless. Such theatrical skills as juggling, ventriloquism and sleight-of-hand were born as entertainment techniques, and these techniques have not found broad acceptance in fine art drama, at least so far. In fact, these skills are specialized techniques performed on a foundation of acting skills such as eye contact, voice projection and vocal enunciation.

The basic techniques shared by the fine arts and entertainment fields indicate that both are skilled pursuits; to do either well requires considerable practice. Moreover, according to the definition of art set out by Thomas Munro, both are artistic, for both incorporate one or more of the following skills:

1. Making or doing something used or intended for use as a stimulus for a satisfactory aesthetic experience. Aspects of this experience may include beauty, pleasantness, interest, and emotion.

2. Expressing and communicating past emotional and other experience, both individual and social.

3. Designing, composing and performing through personal interpretation, as distinguished from routine execution or mechanical reproduction.[5]

For example, the artistic part of stand-up comedy is making people laugh and, when this happens, the art meets Munro's three criteria. It takes skill to write comic lines the audience will find pleasant, interesting, emotional (i.e., humorous) or a combination of all three. It takes skill to communicate through humor one's experiences, whether emotional or not. Finally, it takes skill to perform lines that generate laughter. On the other hand, the Shakespearean actor does not write the play and is presenting drama more often than humor.

These examples illustrate that fine art and entertainment have different artistic goals and draw on different combinations of the three skills to produce their distinctive artistry. Although intended by their producers to be beautiful or entertaining, some objects and productions still fall short of this goal. We have all seen or heard poor quality art and entertainment at one time or another; it is poor because it fails to meet at least one of Munro's three criteria.

Since both entertainment and the fine arts show considerable skill and artistry when done well, we should not be too quick to hold the second in greater esteem than the first. Such ranking is defensible only on evaluative grounds: influential people in society accord higher value to the pursuit of beauty and intellectual expression than to the pursuit of humor and amusement. Nonetheless, people from all levels of society enjoy being entertained as well as entertaining others. Thus many interesting careers in both the fine arts and entertainment await amateur enthusiasts.

The majority of the fine arts have amateur and professional wings. They are found in:

Music
  jazz (vocal, instrumental)
  choral singing
  operatic singing
  chamber music
  orchestral music

Dance
  ballet
  modern

Theatre
  experimental community
  classical community
  art pantomime
  art cinematic production

Art
  photography (color, black & white)
  painting (oils, watercolors)
  drawing (pencil, ink, charcoal)
  printing (stenciling, lettering, calligraphy)
  print making (relief, intaglio, lithography, serigraphy)
  sculpting and carving (clay, wood, metal, wire, putty)

  landscapes
  still life
  portraits
  wildlife
  abstract

Literature

fiction (novels, short stories)

poetry

non-fiction (factual, historical, biographical books and articles)

Some of these forms require a brief explanation. Chamber music is played with a small group of instruments. It includes such solo instrumentalists as pianists, guitarists and accordionists. Modern dance is an experimental form; it diverges radically from ballet in its emphasis on the expressiveness of the human body presented in aesthetically pleasing movements. Community theater is amateur, enhanced at times by a featured professional principal. Although primarily classical, it does have its experimental side as well.

Entertainment is so diverse as to be nearly impossible to classify. Yet one can categorize entertainment along the lines of its fine arts counterparts, since the two types spring from the same basic techniques. The following list of entertainment arts is incomplete, since it contains only those with professional wings holding great appeal for amateurs.

Music

rock music and other jazz derivatives

country music

folk music (commercial)

Theatre

commercial community (musical, operetta, comedy, drama)

entertainment pantomime

entertainment magic

commercial cinematic production (home film and video)

stand-up comedy

variety arts (juggling, clowning, ventriloquism, acrobatics)

sketch

puppetry

public speaking

Dance

jazz dance

choral or show dance

ballroom dancing

tap dancing

country and western

line dancing

Art

sculpting and carving (with clay, wood, wire, metal, putty, balloons)

drawing cartoons, caricatures, animation

photography (color, black & white)

painting (oils, watercolors)

sketching

Literature

fiction (novels, short stories)

poetry

non-fiction (factual, historical, biographical books and articles)

Here, too, some forms need further explanation. The folk music in this list is the entertainment found in various urban venues rather than the native or backcountry art found in the isolated areas of North America and Third World societies. Show dancing is the art of the dance choruses, which liven up many a Broadway show. Finally, the art and literary forms listed here refer to light and, at times, humorous creations, as in funny sketches and sculptures, humorous poetry and amusing short stories.

Amateurs abound in the arts and entertainment fields, due in part to the difficulty of making a living at it, even combined with steady part-time employment in another job. The stereotype of the musician-taxi driver is at least a half-truth. And then there is the joke about the musicologist (musicology is the study of the history and forms of music):

"What do you do if a musicologist knocks at your door?"

"Pay him and take the pizza."

The enormous appeal of producing entertainment or fine art when the job market is withering away in the arid climate of the Information Age opens the field for amateur participation.[6]

All the arts demand a certain routine effort if they are to be even moderately well-executed. The routine is different, however, in the *physical arts* of music and dance as compared to the *non-physical arts* of art, theater and literature. Because the physical arts rest on the artist's ability to use lips, limbs, fingers, vocal chords and other parts of the body, these parts must be kept in tone much as an athlete's. Anyone seeking an amateur career here, if it is to be truly satisfying, must plan on training or practicing nearly every day. My studies of musicians suggest a minimum of 45 to 60 minutes per daily session five days a week for any physical artist who wants to improve. The basic problem is that these artists (both amateur and professional) can atrophy in their physical skills after two days away from their routine. French pianist and composer Robert Casadesus once remarked in an interview that he could tell from his playing when he took a day off and his wife could tell when he took two days off. A decline of this sort is painful for the performer, who must now try to recover what was lost while enduring inferior execution in the meantime.

People seeking an amateur career in the non-physical arts face a different routine. Their creativity flows more or less directly from the mind; it does not require a specialized physical capacity to express it. The readiness of the mind to respond with artistic ideas atrophies more slowly than the readiness of the body to implement them. Thus writers and actors, for example, don't need to train or practice as regularly as musicians and dancers. Nevertheless, non-physical artists are quick to point out that too much time away from the art leads to noticeable mental sluggishness, to a slowness and fuzziness in expressing one's artistic ideas. In this respect, although it is unnecessary to pursue the art almost daily, these artists cannot spend, say, two weeks away from it without feeling the effects.

So routine is important in the two types of fine art. Yet, people unfamiliar with serious leisure activities requiring routine involvement often ask why anyone would want to bother with it during their free time. "It sounds too much like work," they argue. But these amateurs would have it no other way, for it is through routine pursuit that they realize the rewards that come from doing a complicated activity well. Playing around at the activity as a dabblers do is unsatisfying for the amateur (and the professional).

Although in the past some amateurs in the fine arts were self-taught, some formal training is now the norm in all of them. To reach the competence of the least demanding adult level, most novices in music should expect to spend at least one year taking private lessons, whereas those in art, dance and theater should expect to complete an established program. This presumes nearly daily stints of individual practice close to an hour long between lessons or classes for physical artists. Would-be poets and novelists can take writing courses, which are also organized into programs. Here, too, homework is required to improve literary skills. Formal training, although in principle as necessary, is simply unavailable in many of the entertainment arts. In magic, stand-up comedy and the variety arts, amateurs commonly learn by reading manuals, watching professionals and other amateurs, arranging to be tutored by professionals and learning by trial-and-error. By contrast, the Yellow Pages refer to many public speaking training programs.

In general, the fine and entertainment arts appeal to all ages; only rarely do they interest only one or a few age categories (e.g., ballet, modern dance). Still, physical problems such as arthritis, heart disease and inflexibility of joints can force older amateurs out of the physical arts or prevent would-be older amateurs from entering them. To the extent that mental acuity declines with age, similar limitations are found in the non-physical arts as well. But age is not otherwise a barrier to participation. Indeed, some of its adverse effects can be lessened somewhat by pursuing a vigorous amateur career. That having been said, it is a good idea to take up an art no later than middle adulthood, if possible, for novices need time to develop the competence required to perform it at a satisfying level.

Amateur careers in the arts and entertainment fields occur within a sequence of stages. The beginning stage of this career lasts until interest in the activity is established. This is clearly a stage with imprecise boundaries, for some amateurs develop their interests only gradually, whereas others are struck by them suddenly. Either way, novices must eventually invest time, money and equipment so they can pursue the activity on a more or less regular basis, as something they would now definitely like to do, improve at, be seen in and so on.

The development stage begins when interest in the activity takes root, when its pursuit becomes systematic and routine. Personal improvement in an amateur field lasts as long as the participant sticks with it. There is an infinite amount to learn, acquire and experience; even those recognized as the best are still developing. As a career stage, however, development ends, often gradually, when participants reach the point where they can perform with relative ease, where they no longer see themselves as primarily learners or students.

Thus amateurs enter the establishment stage, when they believe they have achieved a sufficient grasp of the basics. Their task is now to find their place in the amateur world, to become established in their pursuit. The line between developing as an amateur and becoming established as one is often imprecise. At a point late in development, the amateur begins to routinely pursue the activity in the local community. This entails finding and cultivating opportunities to practice and perform the art, always limited by the amateur's free time and level of interest in pursuing such opportunities. This part of the career can be stressful.

The amateur career comes into full bloom during the maintenance stage, when participants experience the greatest level of satisfaction the pursuit has to offer. Although not inevitable, the stage of decline is most threatening in the highly physical pursuits. Here, as one anonymous wag put it, "the road to ruin is always in good repair." Though injury can sometimes trigger decline prematurely, aging is probably the number one enemy. Its effects are felt earliest in the most strenuous activities.

Each art form has its own social world, itself an attraction for many amateurs. The social world of amateurs in the collective arts of dance, music and theater is anchored in the artistic ensemble to which they belong: the band, chorus, sketch team, dance company, theater company or puppet troupe. The social world of the ballroom dance couple revolves around their favorite dance floors. In the collective arts, regulars and insiders mix to present public performances, where they are sometimes joined by a professional. Some participants increase their amateur involvement by volunteering to help with the administrative duties of their organizations. Around this core lies a set of peripheral services provided by suppliers (of strings, costumes, music), repair people (for musical instruments), stage hands, make up artists, lighting specialists and many others. Additionally, some amateurs receive periodicals on their art, possibly as part of their membership in a society or association established to promote it. Live and televised performances by professionals and other amateurs are another facet of the complex social worlds of many artists.

The social worlds of the individual arts differ substantially from those of the collective arts. The individual arts include art and literature as well as the performing arts of magic, variety, pantomime, tap dancing, stand-up comedy and piano and accordion playing. Writers, painters and magicians sometimes establish local clubs to present their art and discuss common needs and problems. But, depending on the art, they commonly work alone at home, on stage, in a studio or at some other appropriate venue. The social worlds of individual artists are organized around these locations as well as around opportunities to present their works publicly in bookstores, galleries, theaters, festivals, auditoriums and exhibitions. Reviews of these works are another part of this world, but only to the extent that critics pay attention to amateur productions. Such intermediaries as editors, publishers, foundries (for some sculptors) and piano tuners, though technically strangers in Unruh's scheme, nonetheless play an important role in the leisure lives of many serious amateurs.

Sport

In the eyes of the spectators sport is an entertainment, whereas players define it quite differently. Athletes see sports as contests controlled by a set of rules, where the main goals are to win and find satisfaction in playing the game. In the eyes of the amateurs and professionals who play them, the following sports and games amount to work or serious leisure. The terms in parentheses in this list denote the amateurs' full-time counterparts. The sports marked with an asterisk are those with both professional and elite amateur wings (defined below).

Team sports (professional)	**Team sports (elite amateur)**
football	field hockey
basketball*	yachting
baseball	bobsledding
hockey*	volleyball
soccer*	rowing
rugby	water polo
cricket	synchronized swimming
roller hockey	

**Individual sports
(elite amateur)**
handball
swimming
diving
track and field events
archery
badminton (including
  doubles)
martial arts
speed skating
alpine skiing and
  snowboarding
cross-country skiing
ski jumping
cycling
shooting (firearms)
weight lifting
gymnastics
wrestling[7]
fencing
canoe and kayak racing
luge
sailing

**Individual sports
(professional)**
boxing*
tennis (including doubles)
golf
squash
racketball (including doubles)
jai alai (including doubles)
equestrian events*
bowling
figure skating*
auto racing
motorcycle racing
rodeo (calf roping, steer
  wrestling, bull riding, etc.)

Descriptions of these sports are available in all the larger encyclopedias.

Defining amateurs and professionals in sport is difficult. Using the time-and-money definition in Chapter 1, it is easy to argue that the state-supported elite amateurs competing in the Olympic Games and other international contests are basically professional. True, many countries still officially deny this de facto status, even while joining with various commercial sponsors to provide these athletes with room and board and even money for casual spending. This support enables the athletes to devote themselves full-time to perfecting their sport, much as professional players do. Although professional both by definition and by competence, elite amateurs generally lack the glamor and respect enjoyed by true professionals. Still, these amateurs are highly influential in their own social worlds, where they are considered insiders by the much larger number of regular amateurs.

Since sport is by definition a physical undertaking, a routine practice and training schedule is as necessary as in the physical arts and for the same reasons. Moreover, the minimal effective period of daily training is approximately the same, around 45 to 60 minutes. Finally, as in the arts, playing any sport as a dabbler brings comparatively little satisfaction once the player becomes familiar with the rewards of playing as a dedicated amateur (or professional).

Training in amateur-professional, amateur-elite sports is always formal. Initially, you join a basketball or football team, for example, where you are trained by the coach. Novices in most individual sports typically start by taking lessons from a professional or elite amateur. This is not true, however, for wrestling and track and field. Here you join a "team" of individual contestants, receiving their instruction and criticism from its coach. Some golf and tennis amateurs start their sports careers on similar teams. Rodeo and auto and motorcycle racing are the only sports in this list where you learn chiefly by watching, asking questions and, at times, arranging for regular instruction.

The physical nature of sport sets age limits with the same relentlessness as the physical arts do. But it is also true that sports vary widely in the physical intensity and flexibility needed to play them at a satisfying amateur level. Age 40 is more or less the upper limit for the contact sports of football, rugby, hockey, boxing, rodeo and wrestling. Few people seem to compete beyond this age in the highly aerobic sports of hockey, rowing, soccer, basketball, figure skating, field hockey and speed skating. In other highly aerobic sports – cycling, racquetball, swimming and cross-country skiing – age-graded competitions extend the age limits considerably. Moreover, people in their 60s, and some even their 70s, swim, cycle and cross-country ski for exercise and conditioning, without treating these activities as competitive sports. The same may be said for tennis played outside of tournaments. Finally, people in their 70s participate extensively in low physical intensity sports such as golf, shooting, bowling, yachting and sailing. A wide range of ages also finds great satisfaction in baseball and cricket.

In general, the amateur sports career advances through the same set of stages as physical arts and entertainment. The two careers do diverge in several ways, however. For instance, for many amateurs in sport the transition to the establishment stage is abrupt and clear: they are invited to join an adult team (e.g., park board, university, industrial) or a local club or they are placed on a list of qualified competitors. Furthermore, among artists, only those in the more rigorous forms of dance are familiar with the unyielding age limits to high-aerobic or high-impact sports. Art and sports amateurs have usually finished competing at the most rigorous levels by age 40, at the very outside.

Each sport listed here has its own social world. In amateur team sport, the team itself and its coach form the center of the social world of its members. Games, usually held once a week, and practices, often held two or three times a week, make up another part of this core, along with post-practice and post-game get-togethers with teammates. Strangers here and in the individual sports include judges, referees, equipment suppliers and trainers (for those teams able to afford them).

The social world of the athlete in the individual sports revolves around a particular competition site, for example, courts, tracks, swimming pools and skating rinks. The athlete both practices and competes here, and meets like-minded enthusiasts. In Canada and Great Britain this core also includes the clubs that organize many of these sports and any coaches who work there either for no pay or for a small fee. In the United States the individual sports are commonly organized by high schools, colleges and universities.

The social world of team sport also encompasses the league in which the team plays, the other teams in the league, the schedule of games and the ever-changing team standings. The equivalent in individual sports is the usual series of competitions entered throughout the season, events that are not normally related to one another by calculating standings. Clubs compete in these events as do their individual members, winning or losing against the other competing clubs according to the accumulated successes and failures of the individuals.

The professionals and elite amateurs make up still another important part of the social world of amateur sport. These insiders serve as examples of excellence in the sport. One may be hired to coach a team or a club or, more rarely, an individual athlete. Some are invited to give clinics or demonstrations. During informal get-togethers, regular amateurs learn from professionals and elite amateurs about life in the "big time." To help them perform better, regular amateurs also gather tips on technique, equipment, strategy and other pertinent concerns. Sometimes these experts communicate through nationally or internationally distributed magazines such as *Bicycling, Golf Digest* and *Cross-Country Skier* or through the newsletters of national organizations.

Science

My research on serious leisure in science revealed three kinds of participants: observers, armchair participants and applied scientists. The observers are amateurs; they directly experience their objects of interest through scientific inquiry. The armchair participants are liberal arts hobbyists who pursue their interests largely, if not wholly, through reading. They either prefer this approach to observation or they lack the time, equipment, opportunity or physical stamina to go into the field or laboratory. The applied scientists, who are also amateurs, express their knowledge in some practical way. As far as we know, the most active group of applied amateurs is in computer science.

The amateur observers vary much more than their professional counterparts in their knowledge and willingness and ability to contribute original data to their science. The observers can be classified according to one of three subtypes: apprentices, journeymen or masters.[8] The leisure career of the amateur scientist unfolds from apprentice to journeyman and possibly on to master. Such passage is an inexact process, however, for acquiring knowledge, experience and personal confidence is always gradual.

Scientific apprentices are learners. They hope to learn enough about their discipline, its research procedures and its instrumentation to function as journeymen and eventually, perhaps, as masters. As their knowledge about their science grows, some apprentices select a specialty, becoming learners here as well. Scientific apprentices, unlike their equivalents in the trades, are normally independent; formal association with a master over a prescribed period of time is unheard of. Even at this stage, these practitioners have the freedom to explore their science on their own, although at this point, they are typically can't make an original contribution to the discipline.

Journeymen are knowledgeable, reliable practitioners who can work independently in one or a few specialties. They have advanced far enough to make original contributions to their science. However, it is a matter of self-definition as to whether an amateur has reached this level of sophistication. The amateurs I interviewed were typically modest, even humble, about their achievements. They seemed to sense when they were effectively apprentices, when they had much to learn and when they needed supervision in, say, excavating an archaeological site or needed more experience in working up a valid set of observations. Even journeymen may feel "inadequate" after comparing themselves with the professionals with whom they have frequent contact. Like all scientists, journeymen are always learning, expanding their grasp of the discipline as a whole, and absorbing new developments pertaining to their specialties. The same holds for the masters.

The masters actually contribute to their science, most often by collecting original data on their own that helps advance the field. They are aware of certain knowledge gaps in their specialties, and they know how to make the observations that could close or at least narrow those gaps. They systematically collect relevant data and publicize it through talks, reports and journal articles. Any amateur can contribute through serendipity, such as discovering a new celestial object, but masters systematically seek new data through programs they design (e.g., digging their own archaeological sites) or coordinate with others (e.g., working as part of a team spread across the country to observe a lunar occultation).[9] Master amateur research projects are mainly exploratory and descriptive, however, with the theorizing and hypotheses-testing being left to the professionals. Nevertheless, when these projects are properly carried out, validation of the researcher's status as master follows: amateurs and professionals alike acknowledge his or her contributions, journal articles are accepted for publication and local speaking invitations may be received.

In principle, every science can have an amateur wing, for no science formally restricts data collection within its domain. Yet, as the following list demonstrates, only some sciences actually have an established amateur component. It is likely the others effectively, though not deliberately, discourage amateur participation by being highly abstract or by requiring equipment or training not available to non-professionals. The following sciences have active amateur wings and are primarily exploratory and descriptive. Moreover, each has local variations so extensive that its professional core needs help to cover them all, a service the amateurs in the area are most happy to provide.

Physical Sciences
physics
computer science
astronomy
mineralogy
meteorology

Biological Sciences
ornithology
entomology
botany

Social Sciences
history
archaeology

Reading in a science and collecting descriptive data on one of its relevant research problems are two core activities in these amateur pursuits. Amateurs in physics concentrate on the upper atmosphere or space physics, where they explore radio waves as ham radio operators. Amateurs in computer science explore the latest hardware and software available for personal computers. Amateurs in astronomy describe meteor showers, stellar and lunar occultations, variable star activity and other celestial phenomena. Those in mineralogy study the nature and distribution of rocks and minerals in a particular geographic area, usually where they live. Amateurs in meteorology participate in local weather forecasting. In ornithology they systematically observe the behavior and habitats of birds. Amateur entomologists do much the same with insects. Amateur botanists collect, identify and preserve specimens of plant life found in a given geographic area. Amateur historians nearly always write local history, focusing on their own town or region, or family history, centering on the genealogy of their own family. It is likewise for amateur archaeologists, who search for prehistoric relics and sites of human use and habitation, describing and preserving what they find. In most of these fields, amateurs follow the lead of their professional counterparts and specialize, as in the study of song birds, binary stars or mushrooms (mycology).

The background knowledge needed for a career in amateur science comes from a variety of sources, mostly found in published material. Credit and non-credit courses are often available at colleges and universities. In addition, articles on different specialities are published in periodicals intended for amateurs. Finally, amateurs and some professionals establish local clubs where they may meet as often as weekly for workshops, research reports by their colleagues and the occasional lecture given by a professional.

Even though apprentice scientists hardly acquire such knowledge overnight, they can probably pass more quickly to the stage of journeyman than other types of amateurs. Learning and polishing skills simply requires more time than acquiring intellectual knowledge. As a reasonable estimate, it takes approximately six months for the typical amateur scientist to develop into a scientific journeyman.

The local club, which is often a chapter of a national organization, forms part of the amateur scientist's social world, which is further made up of places where research is conducted (e.g., excavation sites in archaeology, forests in ornithology, archives and libraries in local history). And since amateur science is intellectual work, a home study of some sort is indispensable and therefore another feature of this social world. The master amateurs and professionals of science are the insiders of this world. The professionals play a double role here, as they also serve as the most significant public for amateurs. Moreover, amateurs collect data for professionals, who use them either to generate new propositions or to test existing hypotheses. The social world of amateur science also has a number of important strangers, notably equipment vendors and journal editors.

Amateur Social Worlds

Nearly every serious leisure activity has a vibrant social world. Although the activity itself is exciting, that excitement is also enhanced by networks of like-minded friends, important strangers, local and national organizations, spaces for doing the activity and the people who visit from time to time – the audiences, spectators, admirers, onlookers and others. Magazines, newsletters, courses, lectures, workshops and so forth make up another prominent part of the amateur's social world.

What makes the amateur social world truly distinct, however, is the fact that professionals play a central role in it. In most instances they are locally available so that amateurs can rub elbows with them, pattern their lives after them and marvel at their feats, made possible by full-time devotion to the activity. Although not all professionals are good role models or approachable, enough of them are to win a place of honor in the worlds of avocational pursuits. They may be seen in person only rarely, but their influence is both wide and deep, due in part to their frequent appearance in the print and electronic media.

The absence of this professional counterpart most clearly distinguishes hobbyists from amateurs. Nevertheless, this lack should never be thought to mean inferiority, simplicity or triviality. No serious leisure hobby can be qualified in these terms.

Notes

[1] Jacques Godbout, "La Participation."

[2] Even people employed professionally in a field outside their avocation manage to sustain consistent, active involvement in that avocation. Thus, doctors' symphonies perform regularly in New York, Houston, St. Louis and Los Angeles. A businessmen's symphony operates in Chicago. Occupations known for their long hours of work, including self-employment, high-level management and the liberal professions, were well represented among the amateurs in all the field studies where such occupations were likely to appear. Additionally, such sports as golf, squash, tennis and racquetball appear to make attractive serious leisure for many people with extensive work commitments.

[3] See, for example, U.S. National Institute of Law Enforcement and Criminal Justice, *Citizen Patrol Projects*; *Calgary Herald*, "Volunteers Armed by Worried Police."

[4] See, for example, Levine and Johnstone, *Silly Science*; Walpole, *175 Science Experiments to Amuse and Amaze Your Friends*; Richards, *101 Sciences Surprises*.

[5] Munro, "Four Hundred Arts and Types of Art," p. 45.

[6] In Canada, see the article by Roch Carrier, "What Price Culture?"

[7] Amateur wrestling has no professional counterpart. What passes for professional wrestling is not sport, but popular theater.

[8] This is not an attempt to liken amateur scientists to tradespeople. In everyday usage, these three terms are applied to any field where extensive knowledge and ability must be developed before independent practice is possible.

[9]All amateurs, apprentices included, are aware of the possibility of accidentally discovering something new. But even apprentices observe or do fieldwork chiefly for other reasons, realizing how rare such discoveries are.

Chapter

3

The Hobbies:
Serious Leisure for All

Amateur activities are the most restrictive of the three types of serious leisure. Performing them at a satisfying level requires routine training and practice in art, sport and entertainment, while science requires that you accumulate a great deal of knowledge and possibly technique. I estimate that no more than 20% of the North American population pursues an amateur career of some sort. My experience in serious leisure research suggests, however, that the proportion of hobbyists is significantly larger.

Still, no one can say how much larger the number of hobbyists is, for no one has studied the distribution of serious leisure participants in any Western society, where it appears to have reached its richest expression to date. My hunch that there are proportionately more hobbyists than amateurs follows from the observation that hobbies are often more accessible. Most hobbies are learned informally, usually by reading books or articles, listening to tapes and talking with other hobbyists. Information on hobbies is relatively cheap and easy to come by and can be pursued at almost any convenient time; you need not wait for a scheduled meeting, practice, rehearsal, public match or performance.

Although it can be relatively cheap to start a hobby, it can be costly to continue in it. Some items are expensive to collect, some equipment for construction or repairs is expensive. Some fly fishers, cross-country skiers and animal breeders sink large sums of money into their pastimes, not unlike amateurs who run up sizable debts buying a good violin, telescope or set of golf clubs. In this sense, then, certain hobbies may be no more accessible than many amateur activities.

I have two additional points to make about hobbies before going on to discuss the different types. First, when compared with the other benefits of having a hobby, profits are secondary. Studies of hobbyists show that making money is never a reason for taking up this kind of serious leisure. In other words, hobbies or amateur pursuits are not "second jobs." In fact, devotion to some hobbies can lead the hobbyist to pursue them despite possible or even actual financial loss. Indeed, even if a hobbyist did earn a substantial amount of money in the pursuit, this would be but one reward of many and, by all accounts, one of the least significant. Thus "sideline" businesses, including some so-called "hobby farms," are not considered true hobbies.

Second, some hobbyists fit more than one category, like the builders of motorized model airplanes who fly their constructions. The classification of hobbyists also depends on the circumstances in which they undertake their activities. For example, swimmer one is a "competitor" because he competes in swimming meets. Swimmer two is an "activity participant," because she swims for the satisfaction gained from developing and maintaining her skill, as well as for the exercise it provides.

Collectors

The range of collectibles is enormous, showing a diversity as great as stamps, paintings, rare books, violins, minerals and butterflies. With experience, collectors become more knowledgeable about the social, commercial and physical circumstances in which they obtain their cherished items.[1] They also develop a sophisticated appreciation of these items, consisting of a broad understanding of their historical and contemporary use, production and significance.

When compared with commercial dealers, hobbyist collectors are a different breed. Dealers acquire their stock to resell it and make a profit; their motives are clearly different from those driving collectors. Although collectors may try to make enough money selling a violin or painting to buy one of greater value, they are usually more interested in gaining a prestigious item for social and personal reasons, or possibly to hedge inflation, than in making a profit. Additionally, unlike a dealer, many collectors hope to acquire an entire series or category of a collectible (e.g., all the posters of the Newport Jazz Festival, all the books in the Nancy Drew series).

Casually collecting things like matchbooks, beer bottles and travel pennants is, at best, a marginal hobby. Such items offer nowhere near the same complex of social, commercial and physical circumstances to learn about; no substantial aesthetic or technical appreciation to be cultivated; no comparable level of understanding of production and use to be developed. Casual collecting is therefore casual leisure, a simple diversion. As Allan Olmsted puts it, those who collect with little seriousness are "accumulators."[2]

Robert Overs, author of *Guide to Avocational Activities*, developed a classification of collections. His nine categories are used here with several changes and additions to bring it in line with the above definition of hobbies.

POSTER COLLECTIONS Some posters are issued as a series to publicize a regular or sporadic event. Examples include those announcing arts festivals, academic conferences and community fairs. Other posters announce one-shot events, such as a photography exhibition, sports tournament or program of courses. And still others convey an important message of some kind. The serious collector specializes in certain kinds of posters, including information about their production and availability, about events, messages or situations of interest.

COIN, CURRENCY AND MEDAL COLLECTIONS With the exception of pin collecting, this is numismatics. Overs classifies coin and currency collections into ancient, foreign and domestic and medals into religious, military, commemorative and novelty. The numismatist strives to learn about the social and political history of the items collected, as well as about their production and composition.

STAMP COLLECTIONS Philately is the name for this hobby. The serious philatelist not only collects stamps but also tries to acquire information about the social and economic circumstances surrounding the decision to print each issue. Many stamps artistically express particular customs or the values of a nation; they are also of great interest to collectors.

NATURAL OBJECT COLLECTIONS Overs classifies these items as follows:

❋ fossils

❋ animal trophies and stuffed specimens

❋ moths, insects and butterflies

❀ ferns and wild flowers

❀ leaves, pine cones, etc.

❀ rocks, stones and minerals

❀ pearls, seashells, starfish, sponges, sand, etc.

Each natural object lends itself to detailed study about its formation, natural history and environment.

MODEL COLLECTIONS With so many different kinds of models, collectors have little choice but to specialize. Some collect models of trains, cars, ships, airplanes or animals. Others go in for toys, kites or weapons. Even then, some types of models are so diverse that collectors are forced by limited time and money to concentrate on one or a few subcategories.

DOLL COLLECTIONS Dolls reflect a great deal about the culture and practices of a particular time in a particular society. Perhaps this explains why doll collecting appeals to both sexes. Overs writes that collectors are more interested in antique and speciality dolls than in modern toy dolls, which they consider less aesthetically appealing.

COLLECTIONS OF ART OBJECTS Any type of object created with substantial artistry or craftsmanship – e.g., paintings, sculptures and musical instruments – can form the basis for a serious collection. Some collectors specialize in a particular kind of china or glass work (e.g., plates, figurines), while others collect recordings or folk-art objects. Although some of these objects are mass produced, they are still beautiful and seen as worthy acquisitions.

ANTIQUE COLLECTIONS What is defined as "antique," and hence as collectible, varies widely. In general, furniture, equipment, decorations and other items are considered antique if they were in use several generations ago and seem quaint and outdated in the present. Their strangeness makes them interesting in modern times, encouraging the collector to learn about their use and construction when the items were in vogue. Among the most frequently collected antiques are toys, glass, cars, clocks, dishes, bottles, weapons, watches, furniture, photographs, books and documents.

CONTEMPORARY POPULAR CULTURE COLLECTIONS Contrary to what I said at the beginning of this section, certain artifacts of modern popular culture *are* important enough to call "collectible." These include pins, comics, sports cards and baseball caps. Pin collectors search for the thousands of different items produced to publicize certain events, attitudes and organizations. Olympic pin trading, in particular, has been in vogue in North America since the early 1980s. Moreover, since all four can be treated as investments, it's more than just a hobby for some collectors, sometimes substantially more.

Preparation time is short for collectors when compared with amateurs, for example. Having decided to collect, the novice need only find out where to go and what to look for. Still, since some things are not worth collecting, you need to study in advance the criteria used to identify collectible fossils, glass sculpture or oil paintings. Collectors of natural objects need instruction on how to preserve what they find. Storing collected items can also be fraught with problems, which the seasoned collector has learned to solve. For instance, a dry environment can cause antique furniture to crack or book bindings to putrefy. Only accumulators collect with no preparation whatsoever.

Careers in collecting center heavily on acquiring objects and knowledge about them. As collectors gain more of both, their careers advance, turned from time to time in new directions by chance events and turning points along the way. Stumbling onto a valuable antique in grandmother's attic is a chance event. An example of a turning point is when an avid poster collector is forced to cut back on purchases because the price of posters has risen dramatically. Very few careers in collecting are limited to a particular age category.

In many collecting hobbies, the social world is anchored in a local club or national organization and sometimes in both. Although collecting itself is an individual activity, the clubs provide members with a place for showing other collectors the items they have collected and getting insider information on how to acquire the best specimens of their type of collectible. Dealers (in art, stamps, coins) make up another part of the social world of some collectors. The clubs are important for many dealers, who use them as outlets for displaying their wares and advertising their services.

The social worlds of some collectors also include the people and businesses they must deal with to obtain the items they are searching for. Apart from buying from dealers, who are usually expensive, stamp collectors often ask friends, acquaintances and relatives to bring them stamps. On seeing a pin they like, collectors approach its wearer in hope of trading another pin for the one desired. Antique collectors frequent shops most likely to carry items of interest to them, for which they haggle with the staff to get the best price. Some collectors also haunt auctions, garage sales and flea markets. Some collectible items, such as guns and stamps, are presented at shows periodically. However, many collections are asocial; to pursue these hobbies, the collectors need only head for the woods or the shore or curl up on the couch with a good mail-order catalog.

Makers and Tinkers

Grouped under this heading are such enthusiasts as inventors, seamstresses, automobile repairers, and toy and furniture makers. Excluded are do-it-yourselfers who paint the house to avoid the expense of a tradesperson, whose motives contrast sharply with those of the hobbyist home remodeller. Because they are both work roles and business roles, commercial automobile repair, clothing manufacture and pottery making are also excluded from consideration here.

Although it may seem odd, it is entirely consistent with the extended meaning of "maker" to include those hobbyists who breed or display fish, birds, reptiles and animals. This also embraces the people who avocationally breed or display dogs, cats, sheep, horses, ferrets and llamas.

Robert Overs' classification of "Craft Activities" provides the framework for the following discussion of the making and tinkering hobbies.

COOKING, BAKING AND CANDY-MAKING This category covers a range of activities from making candy and sausages to baking cakes, pies, cookies and breads. Some hobbyists enjoy cooking ethnic specialities from traditional recipes. Others go in for decorating cakes. Additionally, those hobbyists often use special social occasions to present the fruits of their talents.

BEVERAGE CRAFTS Those who make a hobby of producing their own wine, beer, liqueurs and similar forms of drink are classified here. Although books exist on these subjects, kits with instructions are also widely available in specialty stores, which also sell the necessary equipment and ingredients. There, too, the beginner can receive advice from staff.

DECORATING ACTIVITIES Overs lists two kinds of activities here: arranging flowers and decorating small objects. The first is carried out using either fresh or artificial flowers. Using your imagination, you can decorate any small object in an aesthetically pleasing manner. Overs mentions etching pieces of glass and burning designs in wood. Hobbyists also embellish thimbles, washers, toothpicks and drinking glasses, to name but a few possibilities. Decoupage (the art of decorating surfaces with cutouts) and collage (the art of making compositions from ordinary materials such as cloth, paper, metal) are also decorating activities. Creating mobiles and stencils falls into this class of hobby.

INTERLACING, INTERLOCKING AND KNOT-MAKING ACTIVITIES These activities include wicker work and basketweaving as well as macrame and other knot-making activities, of which fly-tying is a well-known form. Quilting, knitting, weaving and crocheting also fall under this heading, as does making hooked, braided and woven rugs. Last but certainly not least are lacework, embroidery and tapestry.

TOY, MODEL AND KIT ASSEMBLY This category spans an enormous variety of activities, from making puppets (figures formed with a costumed hand), marionettes (figures manipulated by strings or wires), and dolls and doll furniture to constructing models of trains, cars, boats, airplanes, rockets and the like. Some of these hobbyists build model houses or furniture, while others devote themselves to electronic projects made from kits (e.g., radios, stereos, television sets). Finally, repairing toys, models and game and sports equipment may become a hobby for those with children or grandchildren, or who have children in the neighborhood.

PAPER CRAFTS Hobbies in this category that appeal to adults include scrapbook projects and papier-mâché constructions (technically a hybrid of sculpture and paper-cutting). Origami, the Oriental art of paper folding, employs a range of skills, some of which are highly evolved. Bookbinding is a supplementary craft used by hobbyists pursuing scrapbook projects and people wanting to bind their personal diaries.

LEATHER AND TEXTILE CRAFTS Hobbyists sew an assortment of products using felt, cloth or leather, either alone or in combination, sometimes embellished with dyes. The most common include belts, gloves, purses, costumes, moccasins and various articles of clothing.

WOOD AND METAL WORKING ACTIVITIES One of the best known activities in this category is woodworking, the craft of using hand and power tools to build everything from bookends and birdhouses to furniture and garden sheds. As rewarding are the metal projects, which draw on the hobbyist's welding and soldering skills, among others. Less common is whittling – wood sculpture using a knife instead of the chisels, gouges and other tools of ordinary woodworking. Whittlers produce bowls, bookends, figurines, napkin rings and a multitude of other objects.

DO-IT-YOURSELF ACTIVITIES These activities constitute a hobby only if approached as leisure. Moreover, because it is a one-shot undertaking, a single do-it-yourself project cannot serve as a hobby, however satisfying. But keeping one's own home and perhaps the homes of friends, relatives and neighbors in good running order can turn into a regular and most rewarding pursuit. Such a pursuit requires a range of skills and knowledge that can be applied to appliance repair, plumbing work, electrical work, and interior and exterior house construction and decoration using tile, paint, varnish, siding, panels, roofing, drywall and wallpaper. Auto and small engine repair also fall into this category, again as long as they are done regularly and mainly for leisure satisfaction. That hobbyists occasionally save themselves money this way does not deprive them of their enjoyment in the activity itself.

RAISING AND BREEDING Hobbyists who raise fish, birds, reptiles and animals (usually cats, dogs and horses) are makers of a special kind, in that they work with living creatures to perfect them according to certain standards. In addition to breeding, these hobbyists may also enjoy training or exhibiting what they have bred. The other main subcategory of raising and breeding is gardening, done either indoors, outdoors or both. Depending on the location, this hobby can include raising plants, vines, shrubs and trees. Some of these enthusiasts specialize in flowers, others in vegetables and still others in nuts or fruits. Lawn care can be a hobby all its own. Any of these may be done purely for display, competition, personal satisfaction or a combination of the three.

MISCELLANEOUS CRAFTS Making candles and creating mosaics from such materials as glass, paper and marble number among the activities in this category. Furthermore, many adults and children enjoy both kite making and flying their constructions in a nearby field. Lapidary work – the art of cutting and polishing stones – is another miscellaneous craft. Some people like making interesting objects with beads, buttons or plaster. Finally, perfume making has an allure of its own.

Many crafts depend on developing substantial, specialized skills, as in using a knife to whittle, a needle to sew or a plane to make furniture. Other crafts, when pursued at their most rewarding levels, require considerable background knowledge. Cooking, do-it-yourself, and raising and breeding are good examples. Hobbyists who assemble toys, models and other objects from kits, like those who sew from patterns and cook from recipes, must have a talent for following often complicated instructions and paying attention to detail. Those in wood-working and metalworking, along with some of the do-it-yourselfers, must also develop a capacity for creating their own plans and designs. Lastly, some of these activities can be highly artistic, as is evident in working with rocks, making mosaics and decorating various objects.

Many careers in the hobbies are based on developing and improving skill, knowledge, artistry, attention to detail or a combination of these. In this sense careers in the making and tinkering hobbies resemble those in the amateur fields. But some construction hobbies with light developmental requirements revolve primarily around accumulating completed projects. These include some of the projects under paper crafts, miscellaneous crafts and interlacing and interlocking activities.

Despite the occasional special requirement, the making and tinkering activities are open to a vast range of people in many different societies. Cultural biases aside, none of these hobbies is limited to one sex and all can appeal to the entire age range of adults with the capacity to carry them out. A properly-conducted international survey would likely find more people engaging in these hobbies than in any of the other four types.

The social worlds of the making and tinkering pastimes are equally varied, offering something for nearly everyone. Many of these activities allow you to work alone, socializing with others only to get supplies for your craft and/or to display them once completed. Hobbyists who want greater social involvement can usually find a club to join, or they can hang around the local shops that serve hobbyists with like interests, chatting with clerks and customers. Some makers and tinkers take advantage of the occasional non-credit course offered in their area. In many of these hobbies, fairs and expositions give them the opportunity to display their own work as well as view that of other hobbyists. Furthermore, since many makers and tinkers provide their products or services freely, as gifts, they're in contact with small numbers of strangers, who thereby come to play an important role in their social worlds.

Activity participants

The third kind of hobbyist is the activity participant. These hobbies require systematic physical movement that has intrinsic appeal and follows a specific set of rules. Often the activity poses a challenge, albeit a non-competitive one. The activities in this category are as diverse as fishing, video games and barbershop singing.

Folk Art is one type of activity participation. Since every professional-amateur-public system is based on social interaction among the three component groups, non-professionals who, as a group, have no professional equivalents are logically excluded from the category of modern amateur. These enthusiasts are referred to in serious leisure research as folk artists, for no equivalent appears to exist outside the arts. They should not to be confused with the commercial performers or producers of these arts. Non-commercial folk artists perform or produce strictly for their own satisfaction or for members of the local community, while making a living in some other way. They commonly know little about the professional standards of their hobby, although they may meet some of them. Having no real involvement with an amateur-professional system in art, the typical folk artist contributes little or nothing to its functioning or to its component groups.

By these criteria, barbershop singing is a folk art. Yet, the best choral and quartet singing does attain high musical and entertainment standards. But they are not professional standards for, as I explain in *The Barbershop Singer*, this art has no professional counterpart. As in the other folk arts, barber-shop audiences are chiefly local, composed mainly of friends and relatives.[3]

Folk artists are a relatively rare breed. Given the isolation of most rural folk (e.g., Indians, Inuit, hill people), their arts tend to remain hidden from the general public. Even the folk arts of various urban ethnic groups seem to be largely inaccessible to outsiders in the larger community. Still, square dancing, bar-bershop singing and morris dancing (a traditional British dance) are not nearly so isolated; they enjoy a certain level of public appeal.

Most activity participants seem to prefer one of the other two kinds of hobbies in this subtype. The *Nature activities*, which are extremely diverse, are pursued outdoors. I have classified them according to one of the main reasons people have for entering such activities. But you can also pursue them for two or even three reasons. The nature activities include:

Nature appreciation
hiking
horseback riding
backpacking/wilderness
  camping
spelunking (cave
  exploration)[4]
bird-watching
canoeing and kayaking
skin (scuba) diving and
  snorkeling
snowshoeing
snowmobiling

Nature's Challenges
ballooning
flying
flying model airplanes
gliding
wave surfing
alpine skiing
snowboarding
scuba diving
cross-country skiing
sailing (with sail/
  engine)
parachuting and
  skydiving
hang gliding
mountain climbing
white water canoeing
  and kayaking
dirt (trail) bike riding
  (non-competitive)

Nature exploitation
fishing
hunting
trapping
mushroom gathering

A number of familiar outdoor activities are excluded from this list simply because they amount to casual leisure rather than serious leisure (e.g., camping, berry picking, beachcombing). Furthermore, some of the activities, including sailing, alpine skiing and cross-country skiing, are sometimes pursued competitively, in which case they are sports (see next section). Mushroom gathering – the sole gathering activity in this list – requires an ability to identify different species, most importantly the poisonous ones. It is anything but casual leisure.

The *Corporeal activities* focus directly on the hobbyist's body, whereas the focus in nature activities is on nature, using the body as a means to reach certain natural areas, to exploit natural resources or to meet one of its many challenges. Routine exercise is a corporeal hobby to the extent that it involves skill and knowledge and is satisfying to the exerciser. Swimming, body building, ice skating, roller skating and the martial arts, when used for conditioning, number among the exercise activities that qualify as serious leisure.

Gymnastics, tumbling and acrobatics are a separate category of corporeal activity. Although they offer a good deal of exercise, perfecting a set of difficult bodily maneuvers, or "feats," is equally important. The same may be said for ballroom dancing. It, too, provides exercise, inspiring its enthusiasts to master such dances as the waltz, fox-trot, samba, rumba and tango.[5]

All the participation activities demand a certain physical fitness if they are to become serious leisure. Even those who sail, hunt, hike or watch birds must be fit enough to pursue these interests for at least a couple of hours. Hang-gliding and fishing from a boat require low levels of conditioning, compared with such activities as swimming, gymnastics and cross-country skiing, where considerable conditioning is necessary. Since flexibility wanes and bones break more easily in later years, many people avoid activities like tumbling, gymnastics, alpine skiing and white-water canoeing at that time of life. Nonetheless, there are plenty of activities to choose from for people of all ages who want to be physically active.

Like the making and tinkering hobbies, careers in the activity participation hobbies unfold along distinctive paths, which require skill and stamina. Both are prominent in tumbling, wave surfing, roller skating, mountain climbing, cross-country skiing and ballroom dancing. The number of achievements is important for some of these hobbyists, as seen in their lists of caves explored, mountains climbed or rivers canoed. Accumulating knowledge and experience is predominant in nature exploitation hobbies. As an example, consider fishing and its rich lore of baits, weather conditions and feeding habits of different species of fish.

With the exception of ballroom dancing and team sailing, almost every participation activity can be pursued alone. Indeed, many of them can only be pursued alone. Others, among them canoeing, spelunking, backpacking and hunting, are usually done with a partner, if for no other reason than help and security in an emergency. Whether pursued alone or with others, most participation hobbies have local clubs that organize group outings, serve as sources of useful information about equipment and nearby sites for pursuing the activity, and hold get-togethers where members can talk shop. Another part of the social world for some is the equipment dealer – the sporting goods store, the backcountry supplier, the wilderness outfitter. Others find their leisure lives revolving around certain gyms, pools, rinks and dance floors. The social world of a physical activity can be considered a lifestyle of its own.

Competitors in Sports, Games and Contests

The chief difference separating competitors from activity participants is competition. Both types of hobby are organized according to rules, but in the sports, games and contests, these rules are stated in rule books or printed sheets and are designed to control competitive action. The sports are classified by team or individual.

Team sports
polo
curling
lacrosse
ringette

Individual sports

darts	ping pong (table tennis)
horseshoes	orienteering
shuffleboard	martial arts
pool/billiards/snooker	dog and sled dog racing
croquet	iceboat racing
race walking	powerboat racing
long-distance running	model racing (boats, cars, trains, airplanes)
target, trap and skeet shooting	handball (singles)

Although the terms "sport" and "game" are frequently used interchangeably, the two differ. The essential differences are as follows. A sport is a game based on one or more physical skills; such skills aren't needed in other games. Chance figures heavily in many non-sport games, as seen in drawing cards, shaking dice, spinning dials and wheels, and the like. There are also chance elements in sport games, but they are not a requirement of play. In this sense, the non-sport games of chess and checkers resemble sport games.

Since they can never qualify as serious leisure, games based purely on chance (e.g., craps, bingo, roulette) are omitted from the following list, although the obsessive pursuit of these can make them appear serious. To qualify as serious leisure, an activity must make use of developed skills, knowledge or experience or a combination of these three. A game can have chance components and still be a hobby, because it also allows decision-making informed by knowledge of and experience with the game.

Table and board games

playing piece games (Sorry, Parcheesi, Chinese checkers)

money games (Rich Uncle, Monopoly)

dual combat games (chess, checkers, backgammon)

Electronic games

computer games

video-parlor games

Knowledge and word games

Scrabble, charades, Pictionary

Card games
> card games for one or two people (cribbage, gin rummy,
> the solitaires)
>
> card games for three or more playing as
> individuals (hearts, poker, rummy, blackjack, canasta)
>
> card games for three of more playing as a team (bridge,
> whist, sheepshead, pinochle)[6]

Role-playing games
Traveller

Dungeons & Dragons

Chivalry & Sorcery

Empire of the Petal Throne

Vampire

Miscellaneous games
dominoes

With the possible exception of the role-playing games, the games listed here need no introduction. Gary Fine, writing in *Shared Fantasy*, describes the role-playing or fantasy games as "any game which allows a number of players to assume the roles of imaginary characters and operate with some degree of freedom in an imaginary environment" (p. 6).

Because they are non-competitive, puzzles and mazes are not games in the strictest sense of the definition just set out. More accurately, a puzzle is a diversion designed to test the ingenuity, knowledge or insight of the player. Crosswords, jigsaw puzzles, diacrostics and mechanical puzzles are popular, as are such "brain twisters" as hidden pictures, memory tests and mathematical and logical puzzles.

The physical conditioning and age limitations for activity participants apply with equal validity to the sports mentioned in this section. Sports competitors have leisure careers similar to those of the activity participants. People who play games or solve puzzles follow careers similar to those of collectors and makers and tinkers. With experience, they grow wiser and more sophisticated at playing a particular game or working a particular puzzle. In addition, puzzle solvers accumulate conquests; they solve a growing number of puzzles, moving up a scale of difficulty to the point of entering one of the puzzle contests. As long as the participant's mental acuity holds up, there is no age limit for games and puzzles, although deteriorating eyesight can certainly discourage participation.

Likewise, the social worlds of sports competitors resemble those of activity participants. Solitary game players and puzzle solvers enjoy working alone as much as solitary activity participants. Indeed, like puzzle enthusiasts, many players of solitaire and electronic games pursue their hobbies alone, outside a social world of any kind. The social world of other games players is often minimal, consisting only of those with whom they routinely play (e.g., the wife and husband scrabble partners, the Friday night poker group, the Tuesday morning bridge players). Still, clubs exist in some areas, notably for bridge and the role-playing games, and tournaments are held in bridge, chess, Scrabble and Monopoly. Absent are such strangers as critics, coaches, suppliers, service personnel and the like, people who enrich the social worlds of many other kinds of serious leisure. By comparison, the social worlds of many games and puzzles are simple, which is not to deny that many participants enjoy the social aspects of these hobbies.

The Liberal Arts Hobbyists

A liberal arts hobby is the pursuit of knowledge for its own sake. People who take up such a hobby wish to acquire knowledge and understanding of, for example, one or more arts, sports, foods, beverages, languages, cultures, histories, sciences, current politics,[7] philosophies or literary traditions. These hobbyists see the knowledge and understanding they gain as ends in themselves rather than as background to another hobby or amateur activity. Compared with other hobbies and amateur activities, the knowledge acquired is of primary rather than secondary importance.

The liberal arts hobbies are set off from the other serious leisure pursuits by two basic characteristics: the search for broad knowledge of a subject and the search for knowledge for its own sake. Broad knowledge can be compared with technical knowledge on the basis of degree rather than crisp demarcation. Unlike technical or detailed knowledge, the broad kind is humanizing. Through it we can gain a deep understanding and acceptance of a significant sector of human life (art, food, language, history, etc.) and the needs, values, desires and sentiments found there. Nevertheless, this understanding and acceptance does not necessarily, or even usually, lead to adoption of these qualities.

Knowledge for its own sake implies that its practical application is secondary. Yet liberal arts hobbyists do use the broad knowledge they acquire: they find considerable satisfaction in expressing it, and this may be an important way for them to maintain and expand it. But this in no way relegates such knowledge to being a simple means to a more important end. In other hobbies and in amateurism and volunteerism, participants need certain kinds of knowledge to produce anything of merit. I reported in *The Laugh-Makers* that aspiring stand-up comics often take workshops, informal courses and tutoring to learn how to perform comedy better. Elery Hamilton-Smith noted a similar motive among volunteer youth workers, who attended weekend training sessions to learn how to provide support for youth club members. Dale Dannefer found that old car collectors read numerous manuals and related literature, from which they learn to tour, show and collect cars and parts of cars.[8]

A third characteristic of the liberal arts hobby is the depth of its knowledge; in other words, such knowledge is more than merely entertaining. This characteristic is particularly relevant for the current politics hobbyist. This hobbyist searches for profound news analyses rather than what David Altheide and Robert Snow refer to in *Media Worlds in the Postjournalism Era* as the primarily entertaining and therefore rarely enlightening broadcasts and analyses of political news on radio and television. Entertaining but uninformative mass media reports and analyses also torment liberal arts hobbyists in art, sport and science. Many of these enthusiasts often have little choice but to rely on these media for information.

The liberal arts hobbyist acquires broad knowledge through active learning, by intentionally seeking the desired ideas. Put otherwise, these hobbyists, instead of sitting back and waiting for leisure experiences to come to them, take the initiative to define their own leisure needs and goals. My observations suggest that this is expressed first and foremost through reading books, magazines and newspapers. Reading can be substantially augmented by viewing or listening to news analyses (the few profound analyses that exist) and film and radio documentaries, listening to audio tapes and live talks, participating directly in activities related to the hobby or engaging in a combination of these. The first two are self-explanatory. The third leads into educational travel and cultural tourism.

The liberal arts hobbies are exceptionally flexible. They can be carried out at your convenience, molded around other activities (obligatory or not), and can accommodate the demands of work and family. Scheduled courses, lectures and radio and television programs sometimes undermine this flexibility but, with reading as the main method of getting information, a rigidly structured lifestyle is relatively uncommon.

The liberal arts hobbies appeal to a wide segment of the community. In addition, they offer a special place in the world of serious leisure for people who cannot or don't wish to pursue more physically demanding activities. Based on the broad appeal and easy financial access of many of these hobbies, they can be described as one of the most democratic types, if not the most democratic type, of serious leisure.

What about the social world of the liberal arts hobbyist? People who hope to become fluent in a new language must enter in a profound way the social world of the people already fluent in it. Yet language is the exception in terms of social worlds. The other liberal arts hobbies have at best only weakly developed social worlds. They are often social, to be sure, but the pursuit of these hobbies is generally individual, centered in reading, viewing and listening. The closest most liberal arts hobbyists come to entering a social world is when, to advance their interests, they take a non-credit course or participate in an educational travel program. They usually do this only occasionally, if for no other reason than to control the expense. The liberal arts hobby of historical reenactment is an exception, however, for enthusiasts here express their knowledge of key events in the past by reenacting them within a social world of enormous complexity.[9]

Self-Interest

Some of the activities discussed in this chapter appear to be in the process of professionalizing, in that a full-time living is becoming possible for more and more participants. This is evident in chess, darts, shuffleboard and bicycle racing where, if professionalization continues, it will dramatically transform the performance standards guiding all participants, in spite of the hobbyists. The professionals will also expand and enrich the social worlds of these activities in proportion to their presence and influence there.

The amateur and hobbyist activities are self-interested pursuits at bottom. People enjoy them mainly for intrinsic reasons, for the rewards and benefits they can experience. Consequently, these activities seem to contribute primarily to the well-being of their enthusiasts. Amateurs and hobbyists may also be spurred on by a desire to serve a public interested in a particular sport, science, collection or breed of animal. Yet the evidence suggests that this altruistic motive is secondary to self-interest.

Viewed from this angle, amateurs and hobbyists stand out against the background of the third type of serious leisure: career volunteering.

Notes

[1]Whether some collectors are in fact amateurs rather than hobbyists will eventually be decided by research on the presence or absence of professionalism among full-time curators of various kinds of collections.

[2]Olmsted, "Collecting."

[3]Barbershop is in other ways atypical as a folk art. For example, it has a complex organizational structure serving over 67 000 members.

[4]To the extent that spelunkers engage in speleology, the scientific exploration and study of caves and other underground features, they are amateur scientists rather than hobbyists.

[5]There are a number of corporeal activities of the casual leisure variety, among them walking, popular dance and jogging, where defined as enjoyable.

[6]Since some people make money playing bridge, perhaps bridge should be classified as an amateur activity. But according to Janicemarie Holtz, a "professional bridge player" is a misnomer. She argues that people who play bridge for money do so as secretly paid partners in a leisure activity officially held to be amateur.

[7]The followers of politics who are committed to a certain political party or doctrine still spend a significant amount of time (and possibly money) informing themselves widely in this area. To be a hobbyist here, a person must pursue a broad knowledge and understanding; he or she must do more than proclaim such and such a political stripe.

[8]Hamilton-Smith, "The Preparation of Volunteer Workers with Adolescent Groups"; Dannefer, "Rationality and Passion in the Private Experience."

[9]See, for example, Mittelstaedt, "Reenacting the American Civil War." Mittelstaedt describes his participants as amateurs, whereas I have classified them as hobbyists because I can find no professional counterpart to them.

Chapter

4

The World of the
Career Volunteer

Volunteering. Is it work, leisure, neither of these or a separate category – just plain volunteering? Although my research indicates that some people have trouble answering this question, making a case for volunteering as leisure actually isn't difficult. If the word "volunteering" is to remain consistent with its French and Latin roots, it, like all other leisure, can only be seen as freely chosen activity. Moreover, like other leisure, leisure volunteering can only be a *satisfying*, or rewarding, experience, otherwise we are forced to conclude that volunteers of this kind are pushed into performing their roles, a contradiction of terms.

The adjectives "satisfying" and "rewarding" have been used from the beginning of this book to describe serious leisure; they are better descriptors than the conventional leisure studies terms of "pleasurable" and "enjoyable."[1] While it is true that volunteers are paid in rare instances, even beyond the expenses they incur, these fees are much too small to provide a livelihood or to obligate the person. Finally, volunteering normally requires being in a particular place, at a specified time, to carry out an assigned job. As we have already seen with reference to amateurs, volunteers can be obligated to some extent, although not to the extent typical of work.

This description of the leisure face of volunteering squares well with Jon Van Til's general definition of the process in *Mapping the Third Sector*:

> *Volunteering* may be identified as a helping action of an individual that is valued by him or her, and yet is not aimed directly at material gain or mandated or coerced by others. Thus, in the broadest sense, *volunteering* is an uncoerced helping activity that is engaged in not primarily for financial

gain and not by coercion or mandate. It is thereby different in definition from work, slavery, or conscription (p. 6).

This definition alludes to the two principal motives behind volunteering. One is helping others – altruism; the other is helping oneself – self-interest. Examples of the latter include working for a cause you feel strongly about or working to experience the variety of social and personal rewards available in volunteering and serious leisure careers. In other words, this is an *intrinsically-rewarding* self-interest rather than one driven by extrinsic interests such as gaining work experience to get a job or to fill a requirement in a training program.

The career possibilities for volunteers have given rise to the distinction between *career volunteering* – the serious leisure form – and casual volunteering. Self-interest likely drives the pursuit of such a career more than altruism, even when people's altruism prompts them to enter the field in the first place. Of the two, self-interest seems to be the stronger motivator, encouraging a volunteer to continue in a serious volunteer leisure career. This is because volunteering requires certain skills, knowledge or training and, at times, two or three of these. Their acquisition is highly rewarding. By contrast, giving blood, helping distribute flyers or taking tickets at performances of the local community theater – all casual volunteering – can never qualify as career volunteering. They require no significant skill, knowledge or training.

In spite of the requirements, career volunteering appears to create no greater load of commitments than many other serious leisure pursuits. For example, volunteers can be obligated to attend rehearsals and perform in the next concert of the community orchestra, play for their team in an upcoming game in the local industrial baseball league, or go to the neighborhood primary school two days a week to help children with reading problems. What makes this free of obligation is that these musicians, athletes and volunteers can terminate their commitment with relative ease. Having met all original obligations, they are free to be unavailable for future projects. True leisure, including career volunteering, contains a substantial degree of choice, even though some people may have to wait to exercise it.

Volunteers working in an organization usually perform tasks assigned by their superiors, who are normally either management employees or senior volunteers.[2] These are tasks the staff believe the volunteers can do, given adequate training and experience, which are either beyond their jurisdiction or, given budgetary limitations, which they cannot do themselves. This arrangement turns volunteers into "outsiders" in organizations otherwise composed of insiders. Indeed, some insiders may even feel threatened by them. These volunteers usually require sponsors, an arrangement unheard of in the individualized amateur and hobbyist activities. In the group amateur and hobbyist pursuits, try-outs provide enough proof of the excellence of a performer or an athlete, removing the need for a sponsor. Organizational volunteers are thus neither akin to professionals, as amateurs are, nor hired workers. Rather they are a special class of helper in someone else's occupational world.[3]

As with other serious leisure, career volunteers occasionally need to persevere. People who want to continue experiencing the same satisfaction in an activity have to meet certain challenges from time to time. Thus, musicians must practice to master difficult musical passages, baseball players must throw repeatedly to perfect their pitches, and volunteers must search for new approaches with which to help children with reading problems. Perseverance can also help volunteers realize their goals and express themselves. In all three types of serious leisure, the deepest satisfaction sometimes comes at the end of the activity rather than during it.

Leisure volunteering is special because it is invariably propelled by its altruism. What makes volunteering rewarding and therefore leisurelike is the unselfish regard for another person or people as expressed through particular acts or activities. Altruism is largely absent in amateurism and hobbies; any altruistic action is really volunteer work done as a sideline to the person's amateur or hobbyist interest.

Volunteers and amateurs do make at least one similar contribution, however; they connect the occupation or organization with which they are associated to its public or clients. For example, Armand Lauffer and Sarah Gorodezky noted in *Volunteers* that "volunteers sometimes speak the clients' language more directly than paid staff" (p. 10). In my own research on amateur scientists, I discovered that they are recognized not only for their scientific work but also for their volunteer work. Here, as unofficial public relations officers, they strive to educate the public in the fundamentals of their science and to lobby the government for legislation in favor of it.

Types of Volunteering

Just as you can pursue leisure in both its serious and casual forms, so you can pursue volunteering. Some volunteering is momentary; it requires little skill or knowledge, but is satisfying and sometimes enjoyable as well. Volunteering in a fun atmosphere to take tickets or distribute flyers were examples mentioned earlier. These instances of casual volunteering and casual leisure contrast with giving blood or money (as a donation), activities rarely described as fun or enjoyable. Yet they are often satisfying, in which case they, too, are true leisure-volunteer activities, often casual. But when unsatisfying, when felt as obligations, they not only fail to count as leisure, they fail to meet the definition of volunteering. Some people volunteer to do something only to find it boring, difficult, distasteful or in some way unrewarding. For the moment this voluntary action is anything but leisure. Moreover, the "volunteer" is now in the mood to abandon the activity at the first convenient and respectable opportunity.

We have mostly covered formal volunteering, or volunteering in organizations. It appears to be somewhat more widespread than informal volunteering, or "helping." Nevertheless, many people willingly lend a hand to a friend, relative or neighbor in a way that's genuinely appreciated. Informal volunteering may well be either serious or casual leisure, although that depends on the activity. People occasionally help their friends, relatives or neighbors even though they (the helpers) would prefer to do something else; in reality they are fulfilling an obligation. These helpers are hardly taking their leisure, for the activity is not freely chosen and may not even be satisfying or pleasurable.

Volunteering for occupational reasons, when viewed from the leisure perspective, is not always true volunteering. Agreeing to organize the annual company picnic, sit on a particular committee or campaign throughout the office for a charity are examples of one type of occupational volunteering. Whether activity of this sort is true volunteering and true leisure depends on how you define it. It is neither leisure nor volunteering if you only agree to do it under pressure from a superior. But when people cheerfully accept such responsibilities and enjoy doing them, then they have found a happy mix of leisure and volunteering in the sphere of work and obligation. Here the personal and collective are joined in a common interest.

Exploring a line of work by volunteering, a practice common among the young and the unemployed, is another type of occupational volunteering. These volunteers hope to gain experience and eventually find paid employment in the same field. Students are similarly coerced when they have to perform a specified number of hours of community service as part of a training program. These activities are accompanied by a sense of obligation or dissatisfaction, and fit poorly with the definition of leisure and raise questions about their fit with the definition of volunteering. Here more than anywhere else, leisure and volunteering can diverge. The students and unemployed workers who volunteer for these reasons are not usually directly coerced by someone else. Volunteer work appears to be a good way to put them on the inside track leading to acceptable employment or successful completion of a program of studies.

Volunteering for the sake of keeping busy, as a replacement for work, is still another kind of occupational volunteering. Some of the elderly and the unemployed explain their volunteer work in these terms.[4] In her book *Leisure and Unemployment*, Sue Glyptis describes Britain's Voluntary Projects Programme, which develops volunteer work opportunities for the employed and unemployed. Participants in this program see volunteering as a way to keep active and maintain their personal well-being. That it might be unsatisfying is no matter, for they expect to perform obligated tasks as they always have, paid or not.

As the leisure component of the volunteer activities discussed in this chapter decreases and the coercive component increases, their fit with volunteering weakens in the same measure. Volunteering as make-work for the elderly and the unemployed and as a job-finding strategy for the young and the unemployed can feel like coercion, however indirect. Where coercion is felt, the coerced activity is *marginal volunteering*, for it resembles work and other obligated activity as much as volunteering. In addition, the voluntary aspect is completely eliminated when the activity is significantly dissatisfying.

The possibility of coercion and marginal volunteering make the common usage of "volunteer" and "volunteering" and the question of what is true leisure and volunteering deceptive. For example, consider the recent trend in the United States for courts to order "volunteer community service" for certain criminals or the AmeriCorps program that provides students with government grants to pay for higher education in return for community service. This chapter can help readers develop a critical eye for spotting the inherent coercion and dissatisfaction of such practices, despite the illogical language of official descriptions.

The Scope of Volunteer Work

The list of areas of volunteer work presented by Mary Kouri in *Volunteerism and Older Adults* shows the enormous scope of career volunteering. It touches virtually all areas of everyday life. Careers can be pursued through formal volunteering – working within an organization or association – or through informal volunteering – working with family, friends or neighbors, or working in a club or self-help group. Some volunteer careers combine both types.

Most volunteering opportunities are of the service variety; volunteers offer help to a specified clientèle. But there are also managerial posts for volunteers, such as the team captain of a unit of volunteer firefighters or the coordinator of volunteers in a residence for the elderly. Finally, a small number of volunteers wind up in decision-making positions as members of boards of directors or executive committees.

Simple membership in a club or voluntary association is not in itself volunteering, not even casual volunteering. Being on a membership list is not an activity. Members who regularly attend meetings can be considered volunteers in that they participate actively in the affairs of the group. Whether their volunteering is of the career or casual variety depends their participation. The secretary and treasurer are career volunteers, whereas the rank-and-file who regularly attend meetings but take only a superficial interest in the issues discussed are casual volunteers.

PROVISION OF NECESSITIES Necessities are food, shelter, clothing and other essential goods and services. Local food banks, the Goodwill Industries and the Salvation Army number among the organizations using volunteers to serve the poor. Some of these volunteers collect used clothing and household items, some repair these items, some distribute items to the needy. Other volunteers work in hostels and missions providing shelter to the homeless. Volunteers also prepare meals served to the indigent or deliver meals to home-bound clients through Meals On Wheels.

EDUCATION Some educational volunteers tutor students with problems in reading, spelling and mathematics under a teacher's supervision. Alternatively, these volunteers help organize and run field trips and extracurricular activities (see the National Association of Partners in Education). Substantial and enduring work for the school's Parent Teacher Association can also be considered educational volunteering. People skilled in a foreign language are sometimes invited to help students polish their skills in that language, including teaching immigrants English as a second language. Organizations such as Literacy Volunteers of America and Laubach Literacy Action promote competence in English for all. Volunteers, most commonly parents, occasionally augment the coaching staff of school interscholastic sports. In some communities school bus drivers work for free and volunteers instruct school dropouts in such trade skills as printing, textile work, woodworking and metal machining. Volunteers also teach students how to repair equipment used in these areas and several others, as well as how to repair the products turned out. Finally, volunteers sometimes teach the repair of textiles, paper products (e.g., books) and products made of sand, glass, stone and clay.

SCIENCE Some science volunteers also help organize and run science fairs and long-term classroom projects in the physical and biological sciences in schools. Others are amateurs who volunteer as public relations officers for their sciences. In addition, volunteers serve as guides in zoos, museums, arboretums, planetariums and botanical gardens. Finally, they may assist in scientific research projects, distinguishing themselves from the more autonomous amateur scientists. Earthwatch, an American service, organizes such help for a number of projects; its mission is to recruit volunteers to conduct research in art, archaeology and marine studies as well as in the geosciences, life sciences and social sciences.

CIVIC AFFAIRS Civic affairs is an extremely broad area, even though it excludes politics, separately considered below. Volunteering in civic affairs entails working in a community-wide service or project, most likely sponsored by government. Thus volunteers are recruited for municipal services, including government-run historical sites, special projects (e.g., World's Fair, Olympic Games, major arts festival) and many programs in tourism and sports and fitness. Volunteers serve as tour guides, staff visitor information booths and work in programs for youth or seniors. They also help maintain tourist sites and public grounds. Some volunteers work at the public library; others become involved in neighborhood crime or fire prevention. Those with the appropriate skills and experience may be asked to write brochures, historical material, even technical documents. The branches of municipal government with the greatest thirst for volunteers are, first, parks, leisure and recreation and, second, social services.

SPIRITUAL DEVELOPMENT Spiritual development refers to lay religious counselling and education, an area as diverse as modern world religions. Friendly visiting at times of death, disaster or severe illness is an example. Missionary work belongs here in that it is satisfying and neither coerced nor substantially paid. Teaching Sunday school and leading adult discussion groups also contribute to spiritual development. Most opportunities for volunteering in this area come through a church, a religious movement or a religious organization.

HEALTH Volunteer work in health is restricted by professional nursing and medical practice. Volunteers with proper certification teach first-aid courses and present public lectures on health-related issues. In hospitals and private homes, they feed people who have trouble feeding themselves; provide company for lonely patients; and help retrain the temporarily disabled by helping them swim, walk and otherwise move atrophied limbs. Health volunteers are possibly most active in physical fitness, where they guide exercise sessions in yoga, aerobics and similar activities. Volunteers are needed for work with the mentally disordered and physically disabled, to help them adapt to life in the wider community. Some provide transportation using specially designed vehicles, like the Handi-Bus. Relevant organizations include the Senior Companion Program, Grey Panthers and Citizen Action, in addition to a number of disease-specific organizations concerned with cancer, heart disease, Alzheimer's disease and the like.

ECONOMIC DEVELOPMENT Nearly an unlimited number of opportunities exist for volunteers in this area. They can fill one of several roles in Third World relief organizations. Some volunteers solicit money for CARE, Oxfam or the Red Cross, or serve as clerks, managers or secretaries. Some American volunteers go overseas with the Peace Corps to work directly with the people by, for example, helping them build a school or an irrigation system, or establish an effective nutritional program. People with the appropriate training may enjoy working abroad for Volunteers in Overseas Cooperative Assistance or Volunteers in Technical Assistance. Back home, volunteers with an entrepreneurial background – often retirees – advise new businesses or help those that are floundering to survive (e.g., Service Corps of Retired Executives, Active Corps Executives). Volunteers in Service to America (VISTA) work to revitalize low-income rural, urban and native individuals and their communities.

PHYSICAL ENVIRONMENT Some people volunteer to enhance public lands, lakes and streams by, for example, planting trees or caring for lawns and flower gardens. Others devote time to improving outdoor activity areas by cleaning up beaches, beautifying picnic grounds, clearing hiking and skiing trails, or removing refuse and deadfall from trout streams. Sports and environmental groups (e.g., the Sierra Club) rely heavily on volunteers to conduct publicity campaigns as well as to lobby the government to stop practices inimical to the environment or a particular outdoor sport. One major consumer of volunteer time is the United States Forest Service Volunteers Program. The American Hiking Society Volunteer Vacations organization does similar work. Volunteers also teach state or provincial programs designed to impart to youth outdoor skills and responsible use of natural resources.

RELIGION A variety of volunteer activities exist within churches. Volunteers organize and run social events and charity campaigns as well as fill lay roles in religious services. Many churches are organized into committees, staffed mainly by volunteers. In addition, volunteers distribute literature and information about their religions. They work in religion-specific information centers (e.g., the Christian Science Reading Rooms), staff telephone information lines and pass out brochures and booklets.

POLITICS Most political volunteers work for one of the political parties, disseminating information about its platform and candidates by carrying banners, posting notices, canvassing door-to-door, distributing party literature and so on. These people are joined by other volunteers at local party meetings where they choose election candidates, hammer out campaign strategies and organize publicity drives. Moreover, it tends to fall to volunteers to recruit new members and raise operating funds. Finally, some of the most faithful and committed party members are elected as delegates to state, provincial and national conventions.

Outside the political parties lie hundreds of special-interest groups run almost entirely by volunteers. They are political in that they hope either to change government policy or to preserve the status quo. Organizations like Common Cause strive to ensure good government, while those such as Project Vote and the League of Women Voters work to generate maximum voter turnout at the polls. In all these groups the appetite for help in lobbying the government and informing the voters is nearly insatiable. Still another genre of political volunteering is for such organizations as the American Civil Liberties Union and the Canadian Civil Liberties Association.

GOVERNMENT Volunteers here work in programs and services run by a branch of the municipal, county, state, provincial or federal government. Volunteer firefighters and emergency service workers (first-aid, disaster relief and search-and-rescue) are good examples of voluntary action in this area. In *Amateurs, Professionals, Serious Leisure*, I noted the trend in some urban police forces toward using volunteers to staff citizen patrols and operate neighborhood crime prevention programs. Volunteers are also widely employed in youth and seniors' programs. Additionally, the judicial system recruits volunteers to work with parolees as well as provide assistance in courtrooms.

SAFETY Volunteers who work to prevent violence and disorderly conduct in schools and on playgrounds are categorized by this term. Adult school patrol guards are another example. The Guardian Angels, a non-violent volunteer organization dedicated to restoring order to urban streets and transportation systems, are community-wide safety volunteers found in many larger North American cities.

HUMAN RELATIONSHIPS This is volunteer work centered on long-term relationships between children and adults or between adults. Examples include exchange-student programs and youth programs linking troubled adolescents with adult mentors. Volunteers serving in the Big Brothers and Big Sisters programs (formerly Aunts and Uncles at Large) develop similar ties with their clients. The welcome programs for new residents organize interpersonal relationships between newcomers and established local residents. Finally, a variety of social services are provided by volunteers for individual clients. These services include battered women's shelters, centers for runaway teen-agers and halfway houses and reintegration programs for reforming alcoholics, drug users and newly released prisoners. Other volunteer services are available through parental aid programs and aid programs for children and seniors.

THE ARTS These volunteers concentrate on the needs of local and regional arts groups. Groups in dance, music and theater often need help making costumes, constructing sets, writing programs and publicizing performances. These groups are amateur by and large, since professionals tend to rely on paid staff. Still, some amateur groups and many professional groups are guided in part by volunteer boards of directors. Furthermore, volunteers help with various annual arts festi-vals, the planning and execution of which span much of the year. Painting and craft work, although less dependent on volunteers than the collective arts, nevertheless solicit their help to publicize and staff exhibitions and write materials announcing their dates and locations. National Public Radio in Washington D.C. uses volunteers to answer telephones, oper-ate computers, prepare mailings, post newspaper clippings, and organize and conduct tours of its facilities.

RECREATION Some of the activities of recreation volunteers were covered under education, government and civic affairs. Beyond these spheres, this volunteer can be found organizing and running different sports club events and unaffiliated an-nual sports events in running, canoe racing, cross-country ski racing and other sports. Adults serve as referees for child and adolescent sports contests, and even some adult contests. Elsewhere, volunteer recreational workers perform diverse functions at summer camps for children and adolescents. Those who work with the Cub Scouts, Boy Scouts, Girl Guides and similar organizations are, for the most part, recreational volunteers. In addition, volunteers work with children as story tellers.

SUPPORT SERVICES The majority of volunteer activities considered so far are formal; each is carried out within organizations or associations. Running an organization is itself a complicated, time-consuming undertaking in which volunteers fill important support roles. Volunteer help is also sought for clerical and secretarial duties. A need also exists for bookkeeping services, which volunteers can often provide. Volunteers may also be engaged to do janitorial work or maintain the grounds around the building.

INFORMAL VOLUNTEERING To qualify as serious leisure, informal volunteer work for family, friends or neighbors must be regular and substantial. Regularly volunteering to baby-sit a child, care for a pet, clean someone's house or do someone's yardwork are examples. Participating regularly and substantially in a small club or self-help group is well-known informal volunteering, as is working with one of the "anonymous" groups – Gamblers Anonymous, Alcoholics Anonymous, etc. A number of small clubs and societies volunteer informally by cleaning up roadsides, helping street kids or developing and disseminating views on the uses of or policies about a nearby park, lake or river. Local chapters of the Society for the Prevention of Cruelty to Animals offer an opportunity for informal volunteering for people concerned about urban pets.

Career Volunteering

It is impossible to list all the forms of volunteering found in any one of these areas. The forms are simply too numerous to include in this book and new forms are emerging at a faster rate as the effects of electronic technology are felt throughout Western society. Nevertheless, the scope of volunteering in North America is clear in the foregoing list. I further hope that the list provides a sufficient understanding of the kinds of volunteering available to allow people to proceed with their own search.

Some of the career volunteering considered in this chapter requires significant training. Some, including many in education, require full certification, even though you work without pay. These areas are open only to specialists who have retired or who find their work too exciting to abandon in their free time. But entry into the majority of these activities is quite a bit less restrictive.

Some of the activities just discussed lend themselves to either casual or serious involvement, depending on the demands made on the volunteer. For instance, a clear difference exists in the ability and experience required to coordinate a canoe race with scores of contestants and that required to ensure that each pair of paddlers is properly registered. The first is career volunteering, whereas the second is casual volunteering. But both types are needed if the race is to go smoothly. Although career volunteering offers many more enduring rewards than its casual cousin, both kinds are common and sometimes indispensable for the same activity.

In short, casual volunteering can be crucial to a larger volunteer project or activity, even though it requires little skill, knowledge or experience. As such it can be significantly satisfying leisure. Yet the nature of this satisfaction differs profoundly from that found in career volunteering. The satisfaction gained from career volunteering comes from the special rewards exclusively available in all three types of serious leisure, rewards unavailable in casual volunteering or in casual leisure.

Notes

[1]The next chapter contains a list of rewards in which pleasure in serious leisure in general and career volunteering in particular is shown to be but one reward of many and, in most serious leisure activities, a minor reward at that.

[2]It may happen, especially in social action and in advocacy and political groups, that senior volunteers in the organization tell the junior ones what to do. Volunteer boards of directors may delegate a broad set of responsibilities to paid executives within the organization.

[3]The ideas in this paragraph were drawn from the works of Floro, "What to Look for in a Study of the Volunteer in the Work World"; Deegan and Nutt, "The Hospital Volunteer"; Williams, "An Uneasy Balance."

[4]See Carp, "Differences among Older Workers"; Roadburg, *Aging*; Shamir, "Unemployment and 'Free Time.'"

Chapter

5

Satisfaction in Serious Leisure

Serious leisure is distinguished by a number of special benefits, tangible, beneficial outcomes. Most of these benefits motivate people to engage in serious leisure; the perceived rewards kindle a person's desire to enter a pursuit and to continue with it over the years and through the difficult times. Difficult times do occur occasionally in serious leisure, which leads to the observation that it is seldom a pure joy. In short, there are costs *and* rewards, and the balance in favor of rewards over costs explains why people become amateurs, hobbyists or career volunteers. Moreover, the costs in serious leisure show why beginners must do much more than consider the benefits. They must also come to grips with the dark side of the activity.

Thus a volunteer board member may not always feel like attending board meetings, may occasionally have ideas rejected, be asked to perform a disagreeable task from time to time and still regard this activity as highly satisfying because of the powerful rewards it also offers. In a nutshell, self-interest in amateurism, hobbyism and career volunteering is specifically about the drive to gain satisfaction and rewards that substantially offset costs.

Throughout this book I treat serious leisure as a basically *satisfying*, or rewarding, experience. I prefer the adjectives "satisfying" and "rewarding" to the conventional leisure studies terms "pleasurable" and "enjoyable" to describe participation in serious leisure where, costs aside, the enthusiast still finds the activity profoundly attractive. Contrary to the popular view of leisure, pleasure or gratification is but one reward of many and a relatively minor one at that.

Rewards in Leisure

The rewards of serious leisure are the routine values that attract and hold its enthusiasts. They are the objects of self-interest; what the self-interested hope to achieve by engaging in this kind of leisure. A serious leisure career both shapes and is shaped by the continuous search for rewards, for it takes months or years to consistently find deep satisfaction as an amateur, hobbyist or volunteer.

My years of research on different amateur activities, the hobby of barbershop singing, and volunteerism in the franco-phone subcommunity of Calgary revealed nine rewards that participants consistently mentioned in all three types of activity. These rewards were often weighted differently relative to each other. There were also variations within the same activity among groups of participants. As the following list shows, the rewards of serious leisure are chiefly personal.

Personal rewards
Self-fulfillment
Self-expression
Self-image
Self-gratification
Cherished experiences
Refreshing mind, body and spirit
Financial return

Social rewards
Meeting people, making friends, joining groups
Group accomplishment

In this scheme, a main reward of altruistic action is cherished experiences. This distinguishes career volunteers from other serious leisure participants by the exceptional number of enriching moments the volunteers experience.

Earlier research indicates that serious leisure enthusiasts not only rank the rewards differently, depending on their pursuit, but also experience the rewards in ways unique to those pursuits. Thus, the cherished experiences gained from working with autistic children are different from those gained from coaching adolescent hockey players. Likewise, self-fulfillment in these two activities develops different skills, abilities and knowledge.

Self-fulfillment, a process known to some specialists as self-realization, refers to participants' use of an activity to develop their skills, bodies, talents or knowledge, to fulfill their potential as human beings. If the participant has developed them earlier, expressing these skills, talents and knowledge, or presenting one's body in a style show or beauty contest, is an additional reward. An enhanced self-image results from the positive self-esteem associated with being a true amateur, hobbyist or volunteer. Self-gratification is the scientific label for pure enjoyment; it is the only pleasure-oriented reward in the list. It is also a main reward of casual leisure. Unusual, memorable experiences are rewarding because they endow people with moral, cultural or intellectual resources. Refreshing the mind, body and spirit diverts the practitioner's mind from work or other obligated activity or from life's problems. Finally, some people find minor, although substantial enough to be satisfying, financial rewards in their leisure activity (e.g., consulting amateur archaeologists, makers and tinkers who sell their products or services, skilled gamblers).

And what about the two social rewards? Meeting people and making friends is about camaraderie, the appeal of shop talk, the exhilaration of being part of the local scene, the sense of being immersed in the social world of a leisure pursuit. Group accomplishment is possible only in such collective undertakings as the team sports and concerted arts; it is the satisfaction that springs from having done one's part in a collaborative project.

Research suggests that cherished experiences are the most powerful and widespread reward in serious leisure. In the theater arts, performers strive to develop a rapport between themselves and their audiences, the delicate emotional communications through which actors make the audience laugh, cry, wonder, admire and the like. This is called the "gift of laughter" in comedy. The singular experiences found in sport, science and theater are also highly valued: the exhilaration of competition, the thrill of gazing into space through a high-powered telescope, the enriching experience of portraying a person vastly different from oneself, the vicarious thrill of living in the archaeological past. Additionally, being on stage is a source of enrichment – the "limelighter role" in magic – as felt by the lone entertainer, the soloist in music, the principal in theater, or the batter or pitcher in baseball. These moments offer a reward that can only be realized from a base of developed skill and knowledge and only be expressed at special times and in special places.

Self-gratification ran a close second in importance to the cherished experience for amateurs in sport and entertainment. This is hardly surprising in sport where enjoyment is an expected part of playing a game. The connection between gratification and performing as an entertainer is less obvious. Both performers and consumers describe the levity of entertainment – its hallmark – as basically pleasurable. Entertainment is, and is supposed to be, lighthearted.

In art, sport and science, where skills or knowledge or both form the foundation of each pursuit, self-fulfillment and self-expression tend to be valued as highly as self-gratification. Moreover, self-expression was generally given somewhat more weight by artists and scientists. Magicians and baseball players said self-expression was a major reward, as it was in theater, where interpreting and presenting a role creatively is an honored ability that takes years to develop. In astronomy, knowledge of one's chosen speciality is the first requirement. However, among amateurs that is only useful if you know how to "get around the sky" with a field telescope.

The remaining rewards are more specifically associated with particular kinds of activities. Self-image generally ranked next, a secondary reward in art, sport and entertainment. It was scarcely mentioned in amateur science although, as Michael Mahoney observed in *Scientist as Subject*, recognition as a valued contributor is coveted by many professionals. After self-image came the social rewards. Group accomplishment was placed at about the same level in sport and the collective arts. Socializing was even less important, with the exceptions of archaeology and baseball. Procedure in amateur archaeology may help explain the social appeal of this science: practitioners usually work together when excavating or surveying a site. Refreshing mind, body and spirit after work was the second most important reward in theater, but was either never mentioned or accorded only a low rank in the remaining fields. Finally, monetary return was either a minor or a nonexistent reward for all amateurs, even in magic where they charge a fee for their shows.

Thrills

Thrills greatly enhance the motivation to pursue many activities. They are the exciting events and occasions that stand out in the enthusiast's mind, the extraordinary, though momentary, rewards. These thrills are special manifestations of the cherished experience and, to a lesser extent, self-fulfillment and self-expression.

Studies illustrate how varied the thrills in serious leisure can be. In the arts, they are the great moments on stage when rapport with the audience is at its peak and performers are at their best. Barbershop singers thrill to the experience of being swallowed up in a sea of barbershop song, surrounded by pure, ringing, consonant harmonies to which the audience avidly responds. As for science, it is thrilling to discover something like a comet or burial site. Avocational astronomers said it was particularly thrilling to observe known processes and phenomena under ideal atmospheric conditions. One of the main thrills in sport comes from playing in championship games, especially if you win. For many amateurs, simply playing exceptionally well in a regular game is thrilling. In entertainment, just being on stage when audience rapport is high can be a thrill. This, in stand-up comedy, is where the comic "kills."

Thrills are also found in significant career advances. They come from being signed (for the first time) by a professional team, opening a show featuring a star comic, publishing one's first scientific article or landing a "plum" role in a major play. Some respondents, mainly young adult amateurs, said it was thrilling to meet a famous practitioner in their field. Among professional magicians it was a rare career thrill to be invited to perform at the Magic Castle in Los Angeles, the private clubhouse of the Academy of Magical Arts.

Are there gender differences in the patterns of rewards and thrills in different serious leisure activities? No research suggests any differences whatsoever. To be sure, some studies were conducted on homogeneous samples of men or women, whereas others involved small samples of women and large samples of men. So it is possible that differences exist. It will be necessary to conduct more penetrating interviews in this area than in the past. For instance, both men and women regard athletic competition as enriching, but they may do so in different ways or for different reasons. At any rate, the lack of information on gender differences may be due more to a failure to ask the right questions than to an absence of such differences.

Psychological Flow

No treatment of the rewards and thrills of serious leisure would be complete without discussing the psychological state known as "flow." Mihaly Csikszentmihalyi notes in *Beyond Boredom and Anxiety* that some activities are so intense and absorbing that they merge with the person's awareness of them. This is most likely to happen in activities that are rewarding for their self-expression, cherished experiences, self-gratification and tendency to refresh mind and body. During flow, attention is centered exclusively on the process of executing an activity in which you feel competent. People in flow tend to lose their sense of self, becoming wrapped up in the action of the immediate present. This state of mind is only possible when the conditions are ideal or close to it. It follows that flow makes an activity intensely rewarding in and of itself.

In serious leisure, participants are in flow when executing a play in football, racing on a downhill ski course, presenting lines in a play, talking with dying patients, playing a game of chess, making a ceramic bowl and the like. Flow is broader than serious leisure, however; someone can experience flow in casual leisure while rafting, bungee jumping or playing roulette. Flow can also be experienced in work. Finally, flow can be one of the routine rewards of an activity, as in sport and the performing arts, or found only in certain thrills, as in contemplating one's own completed work (e.g., the meal of the amateur cook, the quilt of the hobbyist quilt maker, the poetry of the amateur writer).

Leisure Costs

The costs of serious leisure fall into three classes: disappointments, dislikes and tensions. Disappointments are the absence of expected rewards; they are usually born in the failure of high hopes. Because disappointments tend to be specific to each pursuit, it is impossible to list generalized disappointments, as I did for the rewards. Indeed, the only generalization applicable is that, in reaction to past disappointments, many professionals and somewhat fewer amateurs develop a cautious attitude toward their pursuits. They learn to avoid high hopes, since such hopes can founder on the rocks of failure. But even here we find variation from one area to the next.

In sport, for example, it is thrilling to play in a championship game, but bitterly disappointing to lose one. Both amateurs and professionals hold this sentiment, for both fervently hope to win. As disappointing is being sidelined by injury or illness, especially for a major part of the season. Third most common is disappointment stemming from a poor personal or team performance in a game, or a poor performance throughout the season. No differences were observed between amateurs and professionals in this regard, as all athletes are trained to think positively about the outcome of each contest, to believe they can win if they give their best.

At the opposite extreme, we find little disappointment in amateur science. A substantial majority of archaeologists and astronomers, for example, avoided disappointments by avoiding high hopes. Working in exploratory sciences, they had faint hope of finding something, the existence or distinguishing features of which had not yet been discovered (e.g., an Indian burial site, the brightness of a variable star). Amateurs in astronomy, although frequently frustrated by weather conditions, only allowed themselves to become disappointed when rare celestial phenomena or processes, such as a solar eclipse or a famous comet, were obscured by fog or clouds.

The most frequent disappointment in theater stems from an actor's inability to perfect a major part to his or her taste. Sometimes it is impossible to identify with a character. Some amateur thespians cannot find the time they need to achieve an acceptable interpretation, a problem that can also plague amateur classical musicians. As for failing an audition, it is disappointing in every performing art.

Whereas bombing in comedy was a common disappointment for amateurs and even some professionals (everybody bombs once in a while), the equivalent in magic – lack of audience response to a trick – was disappointing for less than a quarter of the sample in that study. This discrepancy can be explained, in part, by the different audience reactions to magic tricks and comic monologues. Mind you, the absence of wonderment after a trick is more difficult to detect than the absence of laughter following a line. As comics say, the silence is "deafening" at this point. In general, amateur magicians were more likely to be free of disappointments (and high hopes) than the comics. Still, a number of magicians were disappointed when a trick "flopped," or failed to unfold as planned. In addition, comics, whose work is controlled significantly by nightclub managers and booking agents, sometimes cited slow career advancement as a disappointment.

Dislikes

When I asked my interviewees to identify and discuss their dislikes in their pursuits, I was interested in more serious matters than simple pet peeves. Dislikes are problems requiring the participant to adjust significantly, possibly even to leave the pursuit. As with disappointments, dislikes tended to pertain to a specific field. The only possible generalization was that professionals have more dislikes than amateurs, as the former have greater overall commitment.

Of all the fields studied, astronomy had the lowest proportion of amateurs with dislikes (50%). The most prevalent was the dislike for members of the local club who had little or no interest in collecting data. They were the "armchair astronomers," liberal arts hobbyists who preferred to read about, and listen to lectures on, their science. The two other dislikes – for cliques and for poorly organized club events – were mentioned much less often.

The disparagement of amateurs by certain professionals was the only widespread dislike identified in amateur archaeology (held by approximately 40% of the sample). The belief that amateurs conduct inferior science was rarely heard but occasionally sensed while in the company of professionals.[1] Amateurs are most likely to sense this belief in the sciences offering the most direct interaction with professionals. For example, whereas amateur and professional archaeologists often work together on excavations, in astronomy, the two types of scientists work separately most of the time.

In theatre, poorly motivated actors topped the list of dislikes, a type also well known in music and sport. A systematic effort to learn the art or sport is expected of all participants. But some (marginal) participants want to play or perform without going through the "drudgery" of preparation (learning, practicing, conditioning and so on). Their inadequate preparation not only drags down the overall quality of the performance, but also spoils the fun of the more devoted enthusiasts, because they are forced to work with undermotivated and inferior participants.

A smaller number of actors lamented incompetent directors. Such people waste time at rehearsals, handle amateurs badly or know too little about the play or the art of acting and staging. Alas, there are incompetent directors who combine all three. A third significant dislike was the "know-it-all," who thinks he or she is wiser about the art and the play than the director. With incompetent directors, this attitude is possibly defensible, but certainly not otherwise. Only two respondents in the theater sample reported no dislikes at all.

Favoritism is a hot issue in some amateur-professional fields. Whereas audition committees now help control it in some of the fine arts, in sports, given the absence of an equivalent, it is the number one dislike.[2] Both amateurs and professionals complained about it. In professional football, charges of favoritism were mingled with accusations of unfairness, dishonesty and inconsistency in the way management deals with players. This is the "politics" of sport.

Another dislike in sport, found mainly among amateur baseball and Canadian junior football players, is the undermotivated teammate. University and professional football are so competitive that such players are soon cut, or benched, replaced with more enthusiastic team members. Additionally, at the lower end of adult amateur sport, I found a dislike for the incompetent coach, with his weak communication with players, ineffective game strategies and poorly developed knowledge of technique. Finally, all amateurs lamented – some stating it as a dislike – the poor coverage of their team by the local mass media. Many felt high school sport received more attention.

Magicians, both amateur and professional, listed as their principal dislike weak acts that reflect unfavorably on magic as a whole. Comics chafed at their public image as happy-go-lucky people who lead a profligate life of sex and drugs. Both shared a hearty distaste for bad audiences in general and for fellow artists who heckle, steal material, drink too much or gather in boisterous groups. They regarded "stealing" material – the theft of tricks, patter, humorous lines and other original components of a performer's act – as an offense. As well, both detested having to perform in seriously inadequate circumstances, with poor lighting, too much background noise, competing attractions (e.g., darts matches, televised sports events), bad sound systems, and cramped or nonexistent stages. Magicians and stand-up comics also commented on the vanity, arrogance, ingratiation or maliciousness of certain colleagues. Some are reputed backbiters or chronic complainers. As for the professionals, they are averse to amateurs who more or less demand that they watch the performance of a trick or monologue and comment favorably on it. Mind you, amateur comics and magicians, along with their counterparts in archaeology, dislike the disparaging remarks of professionals, although the above suggests that amateurs may be bringing some of their troubles on themselves.

Comics had certain dislikes not shared by the magicians. For example, professional comics intensely disliked "bad agents" who fail to promote them, promise favorable fees and working conditions that never materialize, or collaborate with a club manager to establish a low fee for their services. "Bad club managers" commit similar sins, which affect both amateurs and professionals. In addition to failing to deal decisively with hecklers, bad managers offer seamy lodging or require comics to collect tickets to their own performances. As in football, so in comedy: participants must contend with politics based on favoritism. Female comics, for example, feel they are less often favored by agents and club managers than male comics, and several amateurs believe others have "an inside track" to the manager. Finally, amateurs and professionals alike detested being trapped in a contract with a manager or an agent whose judgment and fairness they suspected.

Tensions

The tensions found in the amateur-professional pursuits are the most general of the associated costs. I briefly mentioned one major tension – stage fright – that touches every sort of public performance. Stage fright is widespread throughout sport, entertainment and the performing arts. It is even present in science, when researchers present their work publicly, although science had by far the lowest proportion of respondents reporting tensions of any sort. The only other tension in science – interpersonal friction – was mentioned infrequently in my studies.

Try-outs and auditions are stressful for many participants. Where the aspirants are confident and the competition is at or below their level of ability, however, there may be more eager anticipation than tension. Indeed, approximately 20% of the amateur theater sample indicated they truly enjoy try-outs. They felt auditions offer a great opportunity to strut their stuff and land the part or position. Among the causes of tension, for those who experience it, are stage fright, incompetent judges, patronage in old boy networks and discrimination along the lines of sex, style and ethnicity. Amateurs and junior professionals are more likely than others to be tense.

The audition has its equivalent in the individual fine arts. Painters, sculptors, photographers and craft workers must face intermediaries whose judgments deny or allow access to certain shows, galleries and museums. Career advancement hangs in the balance. Until artists are well established, rejection is always a stark reminder that their work may be unappreciated by those who count. Poets, novelists and other writers endure similar evaluations at the hands of editors. Amateurs and junior professionals may experience more tension when being assessed than senior professionals, since the latter have had their work evaluated more often and may have become somewhat hardened to rejection.

In sport, referees' calls are a common source of momentary and, if crucial, lingering tension. Even though players are well aware that the outcome depends on all the plays made during a game by both teams, they are still likely to get angry over what seems bad judgment to them. But a game is never won or lost in one or two dramatic plays or isolated decisions made by the officials; rather, the outcome depends on everything that happens from the beginning of the match.[3] Still, when it comes to "bad calls," players can lose their objectivity. Naturally, they grow increasingly angry when an official makes bad calls throughout the game (to their disadvantage).

Another source of stress for those in both the fine and popular arts is the possibility that things will go awry on stage and thus blemish the performance. Unfortunately, an unexpected incident can, if badly handled, alert the audience to the performer's momentary loss of control over the production.

Because everyone is trying to create a series of effects, to manage the presentation and impact, on stage predicaments are horrifying. This set of effects is what the audience has come to see. Unexpected and uncontrolled events suggest performers are incompetent, an impression they will go to great lengths to prevent. Such situations also tend to destroy the performance's effect by diverting audience attention to a different reality.

For instance, magicians worry that certain "self-working" tricks may malfunction.[4] Comics who use tape players are concerned that the batteries may run down. As in all theatrical productions, the props can cause potential on stage problems. For example, one actress described how she fretted over the behavior of a dog she had to carry around in one scene.

It's All Worth It

The excess reward over cost – i.e., satisfaction – is highly attractive in serious leisure. Nevertheless, although the rewards and thrills sometimes surpass and always outweigh the disappointments, dislikes and tensions, this way of measuring satisfaction is still circular. Satisfaction was further explored by asking respondents whether they experienced an occasional craving to pursue their leisure (i.e., could they get enough of it), whether they would recommend it to their children, whether they planned to continue in it at the same or a higher rate of involvement and whether they would choose another activity were they to start again. It was rare for a respondent to consider reducing involvement, steering offspring away from the field or starting again in a different field. Many serious leisure partic-ipants want more time for it. Those who have all the time they need are the most fortunate; they alone can find the time to pursue their avocation at the pace they desire.

Serious leisure participants find deep satisfaction in a wide range of activities. These activities are far richer than the virtual reality available via computer software. Rather they are directly-felt experiences occurring in real life by the initiative and direction of the participants. Perhaps this is testimony enough, for those of you who have had your interest in serious leisure piqued by the preceding three chapters, to encourage you to embark on your own serious leisure career.

Endnotes

[1]Lankford, "Amateur Versus Professional"; Rothenberg, "Organization and Control"; Williams, "Astronomers as Amateurs."

[2]See, for example, Hinton-Braaten, "Symphony Auditions."

[3]Stebbins, *Canadian Football*, p. 151.

[4]A self-working trick is a mechanical device that unfolds on its own once set in operation by the performer.

Chapter

6

Starting a Leisure Career

This chapter explores the main avenues open to people interested in starting a career in a serious leisure activity. My aim is to provide novices with the information to initiate and direct their search for clubs, lessons, venues, equipment, supplies and the like needed to routinely participate in an amateur, hobbyist or volunteer activity. In fact, routine is an important career stage in itself. Once the activity becomes routine, once it becomes a predictable, manageable part of your everyday lifestyle, you can then start to evaluate its level of satisfaction. Once it is routine, you can experience many of the activity's costs and rewards and sense the future costs and rewards to come as involvement in the activity deepens.

You are now in a position to be your own agent in creating your leisure lifestyle. This chapter presents the main steps in getting started for each category. The initiative for doing so lies mainly in your hands. As self-interested activity, serious leisure is necessarily self-motivated; success or failure in the activity is largely, if not entirely, controlled by you. You should also check the Practical Bibliography for a short list of introductory books written for your activity. Books, however, normally serve only as supplements for the other ways of learning.

Getting Started as an Amateur

The Arts

This section is organized along the same lines as the categories and activities presented in Chapter 2. In the main, you get started by taking lessons or courses on how to perform the art, observing amateurs and professionals in action, talking with experienced practitioners (both amateur and professional) and, above all, actually doing it. In some of the arts, beginners also learn by reading instructional material. To learn any one of these arts, the beginner must observe (look, listen) repeatedly a great many examples of the art. This is how you internalize the principles used to discriminate good work and, with these standards in mind, you can start setting goals for your own serious leisure career.

MUSIC Private lessons, or more rarely class instruction, in voice or on an instrument are the way most people enter into the world of music. None of the five forms – jazz, choral singing, operatic singing, chamber music and orchestral music – can be performed at a reasonably satisfying level without a certain amount of formal training. Private lessons are usually available for voice and the most popular instruments (guitar, flute, cello, trumpet, trombone, violin, piano, clarinet, percussion, saxophone and accordion) in most North American communities. To locate a teacher, look in the Yellow Pages under "Music Colleges" and "Music Teachers." But since not all music teachers are listed here, ask a musical friend or acquaintance to suggest someone. Established amateurs and professionals usually know many people in their art and can put you in touch with an effective teacher. Other good sources of information include high school music teachers, college and university departments of music and musicians in the community's amateur and professional musical groups. Music store staff can usually suggest teachers for the instruments they sell and rent, and some even give lessons themselves. The local union of the American Federation of Musicians of the United States and Canada will know of many of the music teachers in town. People interested in a jazz or folk music instrument might seek information on teachers from the local jazz or folk-music club. However the teacher is found, you should indicate the type of music you eventually want to play (i.e., jazz, folk, rock, country, orchestral), for once they have taught you the basics of the instrument, teachers tend to specialize in one of these types.

Class instruction is available on some instruments, usually in a continuing education program where students learn by playing in a small band, chamber group or symphony orchestra. Choral training is by nature collective, consisting of group or personal instruction offered through the chorus or choir. Although continuing education courses are sometimes available, most adults seem to start choral singing through a church choir, community chorus or barbershop chorus. College and university students may have access to a chorus or an orchestra at their institution, although these groups usually accept experienced musicians only.

Beginners buy, rent or borrow the musical instrument they want to learn to play. It is wise to seek advice on this from an experienced musician, preferably your music teacher. Except for those playing the pipe organ or orchestral percussion instruments, established amateurs almost always own their instruments. But you will want determine your commitment to this pursuit before making a costly purchase.

DANCE Although private lessons are available in ballroom and country and western dancing, beginners in most forms of dance (jazz, tap, line, ballet, choral, modern) usually get their start in classes. Look in the Yellow Pages under "Dance Clubs," "Dance Studios" and "Dance Academies." Friends and acquaintances who know the local scene can provide insider advice on which studio to select or, for jazz, ballet and modern dance, check with the dance department of a nearby college or university. In fact, such departments usually have introductory courses in jazz, ballet and modern dance, open to all full- and part-time students. Performing dance troupes, both amateur and professional, also have information on how to enter their kind of dance.

THEATER One or two semester-length drama courses are normally all you need to learn the basic principles of acting. The same can be said for puppetry. The courses are non-credit in continuing education programs, but they must be taken for credit, possibly even audited, at a college or university. In the latter, students are often allowed to enroll in introductory drama courses even though they are majoring in other fields. Stores that sell and rent theatrical costumes, supplies and equipment (check the Yellow Pages) may be able to steer beginners toward the classes they need. In the final analysis, however, drama is learned on the job, by landing a part in a play and then working with the director to interpret it. As for beginning courses in cinematic production, they are comparatively rare. But such courses do turn up in non-degree programs in continuing education and in the degree programs in cinematic production offered by community colleges and technical schools.

Beginners in magic, comedy and such learn the basics in a different way. Formal courses are simply unavailable in most communities. These beginners get their start by observing the performances of competent amateurs and professionals and by asking them how they learn their art, organize their routines into shows of 20 to 40 minutes and book opportunities to present the shows in public. Budding magicians can also receive advice from established magicians working at local magic supply stores and from members of local magic clubs (ask at the supply stores about these). New participants in comedy hang around comedy clubs, watching the shows, talking with performers and, eventually, presenting their own five-minute "spot" on amateur night. In both magic and comedy there are usually local professionals who offer lessons. Inquire at comedy clubs and magic clubs and supply stores about this kind of instruction.[1]

Clowning and juggling are learned in much the same way. Local professionals and local amateurs can be contacted directly through their own enterprise or indirectly through an agent (see "Entertainment and Entertainment Bureaus" in the Yellow Pages). The staff at magic supply stores may know a clown or juggler who gives lessons or at least is willing to talk about how to learn the art. Finally, wherever the American Guild of Variety Artists has a local union, office staff may keep a list of such people.

ART Beginners in art can learn the rudiments of painting, drawing, sculpting, printmaking and photography through non-credit courses or credit courses given by the art schools and the college and university art departments. Alternatively, they may enroll in beginners' classes offered at local art studios and art supplies stores. To locate these, consult the Yellow Pages under "Art Lessons" and "Art Instruction." Art suppliers who aren't in the instruction business can normally be counted on to furnish a decent overview of local art instruction for beginners.

Commercial instruction in photography – instruction offered by a business establishment – can be obtained from some professional photographers (look under headings such as "Schools – Photography" in the Yellow Pages). Apart from basic instruction in drawing, no formal training exists for would-be cartoonists and caricaturists. Instruction in printmaking should be sought through non-credit courses or credit courses given in an established graphic design program at a technical school. Instruction manuals in all areas of art are available from supply outlets. But evaluation by an experienced artist of your work is absolutely essential if you are to find satisfaction in the activity and enjoy it. Manuals serve most effectively as supplements to rather than substitutes for courses and lessons.

LITERATURE Aspiring writers should search the catalogs of the colleges, universities and continuing education programs for introductory writing courses. Some college and university courses may have prerequisites, which reduces their accessibility to a small number of students. Although there are books for writers, these resources are limited, for beginners especially need to have their work critiqued by seasoned authors. Teachers fill this crucial role.

Sports

The sports are one of the easiest forms of serious leisure to enter, and most sports and the ways of entering them are well known. Many adult amateurs in the group sports began their athletic careers as adolescents and, although they may have reduced their participation in their adult years, they are hardly beginners when they re-enter. To a lesser degree, the same can be said for athletes of many individual sports. For anyone, then, getting started in a sport is a problem only if you're a beginner.

But, some teams are composed of large numbers of players who joined with no prior experience; these include yachting, rowing, bobsledding, water polo and synchronized swimming. Few adults or high school students are likely to get the opportunity to participate in these sports, even if they live in communities where they are played. Beginners living in a community where people yacht or bobsled, for example, face two problems if they want to become involved: how to contact a team and how to wangle an invitation to join it. Perhaps the most effective way is to hang around places where people engage in the activity: the wharf, river, bobsled run, swimming pool. Talk to participants, ask about the nature of the activity, the ways a person can become involved and the kinds of qualifications you're expected to have. In some communities these sports are organized into clubs. Check the Yellow Pages under "Clubs" and "Associations" or inquire at a nearby college or university in the faculty (or department) of recreation, leisure studies, kinesiology, outdoor pursuits or physical education.

Adult beginners in some individual sports may get started by taking lessons. This is a common approach for golf, tennis, bowling, swimming, diving, archery, gymnastics, figure skating and equestrian events. Lessons in some of these are sometimes advertised in the Yellow Pages. Alternatively, you can inquire at a golf or tennis club or a municipal swimming pool. Supplies and equipment stores often maintain a list of instructors, which is where a beginner should seek such information for archery and figure skating. Instruction in any of these sports, as well as in squash, handball, racquetball, badminton, ski jumping, and alpine and cross-country skiing, may also be offered in small classes in a continuing education program or an equivalent community program sponsored by a college or university. Instruction in alpine skiing is often given at ski hills. Community sports centers, the Young Men's Christian Association (YMCA) and the Young Women's Christian Association (YWCA) also offer lessons and playing opportunities in a number of sports. Classes in target shooting are sometimes available at firing ranges in the area (see the Yellow Pages under "Rifle & Pistol Ranges"). Finally, the Yellow Pages classification "Riding Academies" will help you find instruction in the equestrian events.

A few individual sports must also be approached by hanging around the scene and showing an interest by asking questions. These sports include rodeo, and auto and motorcycle racing. The remaining sports – luge, judo, boxing, cycling, jai alai, speed skating, canoe racing, weight lifting, track and field events – are highly specialized and often organized into clubs (or gyms for weight lifters). A combination of hanging around the scene and inquiring at the club's office are two ways to explore entry into these sports. Equipment stores, particularly those in cycling and canoeing, are useful centers of information about races and how to participate in them. Wrestling can only be entered through a college or university team; this limits participation to registered students.

Science

The number and spread of amateur science clubs make entry into several amateur sciences simple. But finding the club may prove a challenge, since few are listed in the telephone directory. You can find some of them by contacting the appropriate department at a college or university: geology or geography for mineralogy, physics for astronomy, archaeology or anthropology for archaeology, history for local history, and computer science for amateur computer science. In large universities, the three biological sciences are likely to be organized either as separate departments or as subdivisions of a general department of biology.

In addition, the local planetarium may know of the astronomy club, if it does not actually house it. The local office of Environment Canada or the National Weather Service (USA) may have contact with the meteorology club in the area. Museums may be involved with the local history and archaeology societies. Natural history museums often have ties with amateur entomology and ornithology clubs, as well as with members of those clubs whose work enhances their collections. Although they seem to cater chiefly to hobbyists, shops selling lapidary equipment and supplies may keep up-to-date information about the local mineralogy club.

Amateur science clubs are sometimes listed in the Yellow Pages under "Clubs" or "Societies." This may be the only way to track down the local ham, or amateur radio, group, as well as the ever-growing number of computer clubs springing up everywhere in North America.

Getting Started in a Hobby

This section follows the sequence of activities set out in Chapter 3. To get started in a hobby, search for pertinent books and periodicals in the library as well as the larger magazine stores.

Collecting

The first move is obvious in the collection of natural objects. In other kinds of collecting, the collector begins by exploring the shops selling stamps, antiques, coins and currency, or paintings and sculptures. Prints and posters are sold in gift and souvenir shops, galleries and picture framing services. Furthermore, collectors soon learn from colleagues in the hobby and perhaps from clerks in the shops about shows, auctions and good quality mail-order services. Those same clerks may also be able to direct you to a local, regional or national club or association concerned with a particular kind of collecting; these groups are especially likely to collect art, guns, toys, stamps, old cars, and coins and currency.

Making and Tinkering

As in collecting, getting started in the making and tinkering hobbies is rarely a mystery. Most people who want to learn to cook or make wine or beer, would enroll in classes offered either by a continuing education program or a related business (e.g., winemaker's shop, kitchen supply store). It is the same for decorative activities – leather and textile crafts, the interlacing and interlocking activities, and some miscellaneous crafts, especially candle making and mosaic making – except that related businesses are the local craft shops. Hobby shops and continuing education programs sometimes offer classes for budding toy and model makers. There are also how-to books, available for all making and tinkering hobbies. In some of these hobbies, notably do-it-yourself and wood, metal and lapidary work, books are the main learning resource, since classes are relatively uncommon. The public library may carry many of these. These hobbies have their commercial equipment and supplies sectors (e.g., the craft shop, hardware store, fabric outlet) where advice is readily available from experienced hobbyists and how-to literature (including books) is sold.

Activity Participation

Of the folk arts, only barbershop singing and square dancing are generally accessible. Both require training to participate, although the vast majority of barbershop choruses (where most people start) accept singers who can pass a handful of simple voice tests. It is often difficult, however, to find the local chapter of Harmony Incorporated or Sweet Adelines International, both female organizations, or of the Society for the Preservation and Encouragement of Barbershop Quartet Singing in America (SPEBSQSA), a male organization. Since each chapter's name is unique, they are next to impossible to find in the telephone directory, if they are even listed. But this problem is quickly solved by calling 1-(800)-876-7464 (SPEBSQSA) or (918)622-1444 (Sweet Adelines) and asking for a name and contact number for the local chorus. Beginning square dancers need only locate the continuing education programs that offer dance classes or the clubs that organize it (see the Yellow Pages).

Courses exist for virtually every Nature Challenge activity. Given where geographically appropriate (e.g., mountaineering courses near the mountains, surfing courses near the sea), they may last days or years. For example, balloonists must be certified (see the Yellow Pages heading "Balloons – Manned") and so must pilots of planes and gliders (see the Yellow Pages under "Aircraft Schools"). Lengthy training is also necessary for parachuting and scuba diving (see the Yellow Pages). In fact, a majority of the people meeting nature's challenges as a hobby start out with some formal instruction.

By contrast, most enthusiasts of nature exploitation – fishing, hunting, trapping, mushrooming gathering – enter their hobby by way of informal instruction from friends or relatives or the occasional class. The routes to the nature appreciation hobbies are the most varied. Few people take classes in hiking, snowshoeing, birdwatching, snowmobiling or horseback riding (as opposed to the equestrian events), another set of activities mostly learned informally through friends and relatives. This may also be true for spelunking. But many people take non-credit classes in skin diving or canoeing through a college or university. There is no shortage of books and magazines reporting how and where to do participation activities. Depending on the activity, look for reading material as well as expert advice in sporting goods stores, fishing and hunting suppliers, back-country suppliers and equestrian suppliers. Finally, remember to check the public library.

Adults taking up the corporeal activities of swimming and gymnastics for routine exercise usually take classes at a public or private pool or gym. By contrast, ice skating, roller skating (including inline skating) and body building are often learned on one's own, perhaps with some advice from a friend or relative. Body building is often practiced at the YMCA, the YWCA or one of the other "Health Studios" (see the Yellow Pages). Classes are sometimes available through one of the continuing education programs.

Sports, Games and Contests

Nearly all the team and individual sports can be played with at least minor satisfaction after a bit of on-the-spot instruction from an experienced player. The exceptions to this are polo and the martial arts, two sports which require conditioning and background skills. Otherwise entry is comparatively easy, providing you can find someone to teach you the basics and indicate where you may compete in it. Apart from reading a book on the sport, hanging around the scene is a common way to become involved (e.g., pool rooms, race tracks, playing fields). Watch for notices of competitions in the sports and community events sections of the newspaper. Some of these sports are organized into clubs (see the Yellow Pages under "Clubs"), and there may be a continuing education program offering classes in some of them. Finally, you can sometimes start your own scene by purchasing a dart set, croquet set or pool table and inviting friends in for a game.

Starting your own scene works best with the various games designed for two or more players. In other words, you can start your own bridge or poker group or establish with interested partners your own regular playing sessions of chess, Scrabble, Monopoly or gin rummy. A would-be player can also get started in bridge through a continuing education class. If the role-playing games have appeal, search for a club devoted to them. Since these clubs are common on university campuses, ask the office of the student president for information about them. Some games, such as charades and Pictionary, make good party activities because everyone present can play.

The remaining games and all the puzzles are easy to learn and enjoy alone. The beginner need only switch on the video and follow instructions, shuffle the cards and deal a hand of solitaire or read the instructions and start to work the puzzle.

The Liberal Arts Hobbies

With few exceptions liberal arts hobbyists also pursue their leisure as a solitary activity. Beginners seldom need much advice to get started. Since reading is the main way of learning in these hobbies, you simply start exploring the library and bookstores with the goal of building the broad, profound, non-technical knowledge so highly prized by this hobbyist. You should be alert for material with which to augment your reading, particularly public talks and audio and video documentaries.

For people who can afford them, educational travel programs can also increase knowledge and understanding in the geographically-based liberal arts hobbies. A number of universities have non-credit, educational travel programs. They are similar to the Elderhostel Program, which is composed of one-to two-week non-credit courses presently offered in over 40 countries. It and the university educational travel programs are good examples of touristic, self-directed education in the liberal arts which, in the case of Elderhostel, has special appeal for people over 50, the minimum age of eligibility. In addition to these programs, there are several partly organized cultural tours, many of which are described in *Fodor's Great American Learning Vacations* along with a variety of culturally-related camps and workshops. Private tour companies round out the cultural touring possibilities for the liberal arts hobbyist (see "Travel Service" and similar headings in the Yellow Pages).

Unlike other liberal arts hobbyists, people learning a new language, who hope to advance to a level where they are fluent in it, must participate in a profound way in the social world of people fluent in that tongue. Consequently, entering this hobby is anything but a solitary activity. I reported in *The Franco-Calgarians* that English speakers who wanted to learn French began by taking non-credit courses offered by, for example, the Berlitz School of Languages, a continuing education program or a college or university. Once they were fluent enough, some students deepened their involvement in the local francophone social world by frequenting clubs, bookstores, cinemas, restaurants, travel agencies, festivals and special events. In turn, these contacts created a small but expanding number of French-language friendships, acquaintanceships and network connections. For some, those contacts also led to volunteer opportunities with one or two francophone services in Calgary. Other students with more time and money achieved the same end by participating in a francophone social world in Quebec or France.

Entering Volunteer Work

Volunteer work is the easiest to enter into of the three types of serious leisure. You need only select one of the areas listed in Chapter 4 and contact one of the organizations to see if they need the sort of help you can provide. In many instances, little advance preparation is necessary, since most organizations have specialized roles to fill and prefer to conduct their own training.

But there are some important fragments of advice to add. First, nearly every city has some sort of central clearinghouse for volunteers, an organization to which people may go for information on the groups and organizations that need volunteers. These agencies are usually called "volunteer centers" or "voluntary action centers." Moreover, most community newspapers publish a section detailing the volunteer needs of any organization in the area. Community radio and television stations sometimes offer a similar service. As well, at least three national clearinghouses for volunteers exist in the United States. One of them – VOLUNTEER – The National Center – was formed to maintain an electronic data bank on volunteers and their skills; this information is matched with the needs of non-profit organizations. The Internet Nonprofit Center runs a bulletin board with volunteer opportunities, while the Contact Center Network maintains an updated description of non-profit organizations. Similar services operate in Canada, including Charity Village and the Canadian Non-Profit Resource Network. Finally, self-help volunteer data banks exist as well; their aim is to organize specialized services for the members of particular demographic categories as rendered by the members themselves (e.g., women, Roman Catholics, the elderly, ethnic groups). The American Association of Retired Persons (AARP) also offers volunteer services to certain categories of clients younger than 50, the minimum age for AARP membership. The members of AARP supply these services.

Getting Started in the Information Age

The electronic revolution has made it possible to develop data banks of volunteers and match their skills with the needs of non-profit organizations. Using a national agency with a volunteer data bank, local volunteers can now make contact with local organizations in need of their help. In some cities the local volunteer center maintains a computerized volunteer bank covering the metropolitan area.

Whether they are beginners or old hands seeking a change, amateurs, hobbyists and career volunteers can now use their personal computers to explore leisure and volunteer organizations for new forms of serious leisure or new ways of finding satisfaction in their serious leisure activity. By subscribing to one of the commercial Internet providers (e.g., Prodigy, CompuServe, America Online), they can gain access to the World-Wide Web (WWW). Here, using any search engine, you enter the name of an activity and then follow the instructions on the screen. This will lead quickly to the (often quite long) list of "documents" currently available on that activity. Since the WWW is continuously expanding and changing, it is pointless to list any Web addresses in this book as they will likely become obsolete. But it takes little time for someone to locate a form of serious leisure on the Internet and read the latest information about it.

Endnotes

[1]Schools have been established for training professional performers in magic, clowning, stand-up comedy, and the various circus arts. Besides being for future professionals only, they are inaccessible for the most part, located in but two or three cities in all of North America.

Chapter

7

Lifestyle, Identity and Leisure Marginality

This chapter bears on four important community-centered issues touching the lives of serious leisure participants: leisure lifestyle and identity, leisure as a central life interest, social marginality in serious leisure and serious leisure in the community. In this chapter I seek to answer the question raised by many of the amateurs, hobbyists and volunteers I have interviewed over the years: who am I, with my serious leisure interest and its day-to-day expression, vis-à-vis the majority of people in my community whose leisure interests are casual?

Lifestyle and Identity

Dictionaries define lifestyle as simply a way of living, which is for the most part circular and of little use in this chapter. Social science definitions have advanced well beyond this:

> A lifestyle is a distinctive set of shared patterns of behavior organized around a set of coherent interests or social conditions or both. Participants explain and justify these patterns with a set of related values, attitudes, and orientations which, under certain conditions, become the basis for a separate, common identity.[1]

This definition refers exclusively to group lifestyles. This restriction doesn't deny the existence of idiosyncratic, highly personal, lifestyles led by recluses, workaholics, people suffering from acute mental disorder and other loners. Rather it recognizes that, to this point, the study of lifestyles has concentrated almost entirely on shared patterns of tangible behavior, leaving us with little information about individual lifestyles.[2]

According to the foregoing definition, some lifestyles serve to identify their participants. In other words, some people are members of a category of humankind who recognize themselves and, to some extent, are recognized by the larger community for the distinctive life they lead. Prostitutes, beach habitues, travelling sales people and the elderly in seniors' homes are identifiable in many ways, possibly the most visible being their unusual lifestyles. The same can be said for the enthusiasts pursuing many of the serious leisure activities.

A profound lifestyle awaits anyone who routinely pursues a serious leisure career in, say, amateur theater, volunteer work with the mentally handicapped or the hobby of model railroading or of mountain climbing. This person may also find exciting lifestyles in such casual pastimes as socializing in hot tubs and "whooping it up" at weekend beer parties. But many other forms of casual leisure, for example sun tanning or strolling in the park, are often not shared with others and are not lifestyles according to the social science definition. Moreover, in themselves, these activities are too superficial and unremarkable to foster a lifestyle.

Central Life Interest

Lifestyles can also be viewed as behavioral expressions of peoples' central life interests in complicated, absorbing, satisfying activities. In his book *Central Life Interests*, Robert Dubin observes that such an interest is "that portion of a person's total life in which energies are invested in both physical/intellectual activities and in positive emotional states." Sociologically, a central life interest is often associated with a major role in life. Since they can only emerge from positive emotional states, central life interests are never obsessive and compulsive activities.

Dubin's examples make it clear that either work or serious leisure can become a central life interest:

> A workaholic is an individual who literally lives and breathes an occupation or profession. Work hours know no limits, and off-work hours are usually filled with work-related concerns. Nothing pleases a workaholic more than to be working. Such an individual has a CLI [central life interest] in work.[3]

> A dedicated amateur or professional athlete will devote much more time and concentration to training than will be invested in actual competition. Over and over again athletes will practice their skills, hoping to bring themselves to a peak of performance. Even though practicing may be painful, the ultimate competitive edge produced by practice far outweighs

in satisfaction and pride any aches and pains of preparation. Such people make their athletic life their CLI.

A committed gardener, stamp collector, opera buff, jet setter, cook, housewife, mountain climber, bird watcher, computer "hacker," novel reader, fisherman, or gambler (and you can add many more to the list from your own experiences) are all usually devoted to their activity as a central life interest. Give such individuals a chance to talk freely about themselves and they will quickly reveal their CLI through fixation on the subject and obvious emotional fervor with which they talk about it.

These are hobbyist and amateur activities. But career volunteers find a lively central life interest in their pursuits, too:

In American politics, and probably the politics of most Western countries, groups increasingly enter political life with a single issue as their rallying point. That single issue may be taxes, abortion, women's rights, the environment, consumerism, conservatism, or civil rights, and much activity and emotion is invested in "the movement." Adherents come to view themselves as personifying "good guys" who rally around a movement's single issue, making their movement their CLI.

In the Information Age, with its dwindling employment opportunities, people will find more and more that the only kinds of central life interests open to them are serious leisure activities. Additionally, employed people will find themselves with a choice never before encountered in the history of work in the industrial world: whether to make their 25-hour-a-week job their central life interest or turn to a serious leisure activity because their job is too insubstantial to invest positive emotional, physical and intellectual energy in it. Of course, for the unemployed and the retired, serious leisure is their only recourse if they are to have any central life interests whatsoever. There will always be people with sufficient time, energy and opportunity to sustain more than one central life interest.

A leisure identity develops along with a person's leisure-based central life interest. In other words, your leisure lifestyle expresses your central life interest and forms your personal and community identity as someone who enjoys that activity. In the jobless or relatively jobless future, serious leisure will be the only area in life where people can develop an identity expressing their distinctive personal qualities. (These qualities are expressed in realizing the rewards and benefits discussed earlier.) Moreover, leisure will be the only remaining area where people can find a community role that can foster significant self-respect. Given the importance of work in Western society, most casual leisure activities, with their strong happiness appeal, are usually dismissed as contributing little to peoples' self-respect.

Leisure Marginality

Each study I undertake on amateurs, hobbyists and career volunteers adds weight to the idea that, at least at present, they, and sometimes their activities, are socially marginal. This is most evident for amateurs, who are neither dabblers nor professionals. But all serious leisure is characterized by a significant commitment as expressed in regimentation and systematization. This commitment is measured by sizeable investments of time, energy and emotion. This marginalizes serious leisure participants in a world dominated by casual leisure, producing a picture that runs counter to common sense. For example, participants in serious leisure pursue their activities with such passion and earnestness that Erving Goffman was led to describe them as "quietly disaffiliated deviants."[4] The remarks of journalist Charles Gordon further demonstrate the popular attitude:

> In the first place, the reaction of many people to the Age of Leisure is to work longer and harder – in other words to refuse to participate in it. In the second place, others have taken to the Age of Leisure by turning leisure into work.
>
> You have only to set foot – or wheel – upon one of our bicycle paths to appreciate the point. For many people, the bicycle is not a leisure vehicle, used to tootle in a leisurely way through the greenery of the capital. No, it is an instrument of performance – used to create fitness, and to measure it in kilometres per hour, in distance travelled.
>
> The bicycle is not to be taken lightly. Bicycling is serious business. Do not go slowly in front of a serious cyclist.
>
> Something similar is happening to bird-watching, a pursuit that used to be confined to slightly dotty denizens of the slow lane. There could be no activity less intense than strolling through the woods carrying a book and a set of binoculars.
>
> Now something has happened. In the Age of Leisure, bird-watching is called birding and birding has become competitive. Last month something called the World Series of Birding

was [held] in New Jersey. There were 46 teams and heaven knows how many birds.

Which brings us to gardening. . . .[5]

Furthermore, serious leisure tends to be uncontrollable; it kindles in people a desire to do it beyond the time and money available for it. Some casual leisure can also be uncontrollable, but the marginality of serious leisure enthusiasts implies the presence of a stronger tendency in this direction. Finally, amateurs, who are peripheral members of the profession on which they model their activities, are still judged by the standards of that same profession.

The marginality under consideration here differs from that afflicting the "marginal man," a concept used by sociologists to explain the lifestyles of immigrants. The latter are marginal because they are often caught between two cultures. Although both types of marginality center on peripheral, ambiguous social status, leisure marginality is hardly as pervasive as cultural. Rather, leisure marginality is a segmented and limited marginality associated with uncommon central life interests.

In leisure and ethnic marginality, marginal people, as well as the wider community, are *ambiguous*, lack clarity as to who they really are and what they really do. The studies I conducted on amateurs and hobbyists revealed the multifaceted nature of this ambiguity. On the cultural side, ambiguity is a conflict of expectations and of values. On the social side, incongruent status arrangements develop, such as when amateurs with leisure goals help professionals reach their work goals. On the psychological side, practitioners may become ambivalent toward their serious leisure as they experience their own marginality. The following episode taken from the baseball study is an example of the psychological ambiguity in serious leisure:

> One father arrived at a late Sunday afternoon practice with his two young boys: "My wife had to be away this afternoon," he commented. "She said you watch them or stay home." He had to leave the field several times during the workout to break up a fight between them or soothe a minor injury incurred while scampering around the bleachers or surrounding area.

In summing up these ideas about ambiguity, both the practitioners of a serious leisure activity and members of the larger community are inclined to see it as marginal to the main foci of the social institutions of work, family and leisure.

My research in serious leisure shows further that family and work and even other leisure activities pull many serious leisure practitioners in two, if not three, directions at once, making time demands that together often exceed the total available hours. Moreover, unlike family and work activities where institutional supports sustain serious involvement, such support is absent in leisure. For example, such widely-accepted values as providing for one's family, working hard on the job and being family centered – all of which help justify our efforts in these spheres – are simply lacking in most serious leisure.[6] In addition, their importance in family and work threatens amateur involvement by devaluing the latter while raising the value of the former.

Most critical, however, is the observation that serious leisure practitioners are marginal even to leisure itself. In other words, implicitly or explicitly, they reject the values, attitudes and patterns of behavior that make up the core of modern leisure, which are mostly casual activities. For instance, many interviewees told me about their lack of interest in television or in such passive leisure as light conversation and people watching. Those who go in for serious leisure lack key institutional supports for their goals as well as for how they reach them.

Marginal status is common in industrial societies where rapid social change gives birth to new forms of work and leisure. Still, as time passes, certain forms do become less ambiguous and marginal.[7] A few of them even become central. Still, according to the research, such a transformation has so far failed to occur for any of the serious leisure activities. Yet, as the Information Age unfolds and work continues to decline in significance and availability, leisure could well come to occupy a more prominent place in community life than before. Such a rise in stature is especially likely for volunteering, poised to take over many functions once filled by paid work.

In the meantime, serious leisure participants seem quite undisturbed by the marginality of their activities. They see them as harmless social differences of which they are rather proud: they are committed to a fulfilling serious leisure activity when most people are committed only to the search for pure fun, even while most people don't understand the values and motives that explain and justify their love for their activity.

Serious Leisure in the Community

Yet serious leisure does make many significant contributions to the community. One, through the social worlds it generates, serious leisure offers a sense of belonging and participation for strangers, tourists, regulars and insiders. This stood out in every study I have conducted, which centered almost entirely on regulars and insiders, however. It also shows in Robin Mittelstaedt's detailed description of the same four types who participate in American Civil War reenactments.[8]

Serious leisure can also stand as evidence for the people who do not pursue it that leisure can be more than pure fun-seeking or a wretched malady of contemporary Western civilization, the bitter indictment made by Ralph Glasser in *Leisure: Penalty or Prize?*

Serious leisure can contribute significantly to communal and even societal integration. For example, Thompson found that the members of a women's tennis association in Australia, who met weekly for matches, came from a range of different social classes and age groups.[9] In a similar vein, to observe francophone volunteers, I sat on the board of directors of a French-language community organization composed of a realtor, a teacher, a banker, a homemaker, a data analyst, a business executive, a high school student and myself, a sociologist and university professor. There was also a nearly equal representation of both sexes who, together, ranged in age from 16 to around 65. Likewise, Allan Olmsted describes how gun collectors from the city and surrounding areas rub elbows periodically at various "gun shows" where they display their collections for the general public and dealers.[10]

Serious leisure also has a positive effect on the general welfare of the community: it benefits the public in important ways, as when a community orchestra gives a performance or the local astronomical society hosts a "star night." Ruth Finnegan in *The Hidden Musicians* describes the complex, positive effect on the different music publics of the entire local amateur-professional-hobbyist music scene in the English town of Milton Keynes.

Given that serious leisure makes many contributions to the community, it can be compared with voluntary simplicity. In a book by the same title, Duane Elgin writes that, among other things, voluntary simplicity is a way of living that accepts the responsibility for developing our human potentials, as well as for contributing to the well-being of the world of which we are an inseparable part; a paring back of the superficial aspects of our lives so as to allow more time and energy to develop the heartfelt aspects of our lives.

The voluntary simplicity movement, also called simple living and creative simplicity, was launched in the mid-1930s with an article written by Richard Gregg.[11] Since its believers also espouse many other principles, this way of living is not identical with serious leisure. Nevertheless, the two both encourage and foster personal development through realizing individual human potential and contributing to the welfare of the wider community.

Finding Organizational Roots

The work – or more accurately, non-work – situation of many people in the Information Age will consist, in part, of floating without a rudder in an organizationless sea, a result of being unemployed, retired, or a temporary consultant or limited-term contractual worker. This absence of organizational ties will likely pose little or no problem for some people; their family relationships and friendship networks are all they will ever want. Others, however, may miss belonging to a collective with greater public visibility than networks and relationships have. If this is true, being cut off from the sense of belonging they once enjoyed at work will inspire these former employees to search for other organizations that can replace this loss.

Although there are forms of serious leisure with little or no organizational structure, notably the liberal arts hobbies, the vast majority are the opposite. People seeking new organizational ties can find elaborate social worlds in clubs, associations, commercial dealers, useful services, organized routine events, and so on. Volunteers almost always work in an organization of some kind. The main exceptions are volunteers in a social movement so new that a formal organizational structure has yet to evolve.

In addition, although there is no arguing that serious leisure and its enthusiasts are marginal, this may enhance their sense of organizational belonging. When the larger community sees them as quaint, eccentric or merely different, their solidarity is strengthened by this public evaluation they must all live with.

In the meantime, many organizations provide socially visible rallying points for their members as well as outlets for the central life interests they share. Furthermore, a club, team, orchestra or society commonly serves as the hub of the lifestyle of the enthusiasts pursuing the activity.

Serious leisure can offer many benefits in the jobless future. But several nagging questions remain to be answered. How can we make the transition to a society where serious leisure will be a common central life interest in a rich and satisfying lifestyle that offers an appealing identity? How can people live if they only work part-time or not at all? Can society survive if work becomes secondary in importance and the main identities, central life interests, significant lifestyles and opportunities for organizational membership shift to the leisure sphere of life?

Notes

[1]This is a paraphrase of my own definition of lifestyle, which draws on the ideas of Veal, Sobel and Bellah. See Stebbins, "Lifestyle as a Generic Concept in Ethnographic Research"; Veal, "The Concept of Lifestyle"; Sobel, *Lifestyle and Social Structure*; Bellah et al., *Habits of the Heart*.

[2]Veal, A.J., "The Concept of Lifestyle."

[3]This is an accurate portrayal of the concept of workaholic as originally set out by Marilyn Machlowitz in *Workaholics*. Perhaps because of the label itself, misinterpretations of her ideas have resulted in the popular notion that such people are driven obsessives.

[4]As good a descriptor as "quietly disaffiliated" is, Goffman's decision to classify such people as deviant fails to square with the serious leisure participants' views of themselves and, for that matter, with the canons of deviance theory (e.g., Stebbins, *Tolerable Differences*, pp. 2-7).

[5]Gordon, "Another Major Step Forward."

[6]Some fields of career volunteering, rooted as they are in altruism, may be shown in future research to have a higher degree of community support than is given to amateur and hobbyist activities.

[7]Rosenthal's study of chiropractors exemplifies this possibility. See Rosenthal, "Marginal or Mainstream."

[8]Mittelstaedt, "Reenacting the American Civil War."

[9]Thompson, "'Mum's Tennis Day.'"

[10]Olmsted, "Morally Controversial Leisure."

[11]Gregg, "Voluntary Simplicity." See Elgin, *Voluntary Simplicity*, pp. 297-298, for bibliographic information on the several reprinted versions of this article.

8

Serious Leisure in a World without Work

For those currently lacking a work-based central life interest, it is unfortunate that, at present, the world I just described is more a tantalizing vision than an imminent reality, because of several substantial obstacles, some personal, others social and economic. Let us turn to the personal obstacles first.

Is Leisure Desirable?

Donald Reid and Roger Mannell, in their review of the research on whether leisure is desirable, found that many people in industrialized countries are ambivalent toward it.

> A fundamental ideology of industrial society has been the idea of work centrality. . . . Work in the mature capitalist society is comprised mainly of paid employment. In order to maintain an adequate supply of labor, including a sufficient pool of unemployed who are ready to replace those who become too expensive to their employers, workers have been led to believe that paid work is not only noble but the very essence of life. People without paid work come to believe that their lives are incomplete, lacking in self-worth and individual dignity. . . . Traditionally, work is seen as the activity through which an individual's self-identity is created and sustained. The centrality of work is viewed to be the major ingredient for constructing social and psychological as well as economic well-being.[1]

Work has taken precedence over leisure in modern times, although it appears to dominate more in North America than in Europe. This is true because people generally like work, identify with it, need the money, hardly know how to use their time after work or because of a combination of these factors and possibly others.

But Reid and Mannell, among others, cite evidence that, during the last two decades of the 20th century, work has been declining as a central life interest, replaced by leisure as the more attractive alternative. This transformation is still only partial, however. Aronowitz and DiFazio write in *The Jobless Future* that "work remains the fulcrum of our cultural aspirations – among them the values of success, well-being, [and] self-worth." The attitude of the unemployed supports this observation. Unemployment revolves much more around the search for work than around the search for leisure; it does not automatically result in leisure, but in free time, time after work. Unemployment is *forced* free time and it has raised the question in social science circles of whether a person in such circumstances can find stimulating, or true, leisure of any kind, be it casual or serious.

The evidence suggests that people experience unemployment differently and turn to different activities to counteract its worst effects.[2] For instance, the unemployed in the upper-level occupations, including unemployed professionals, are more likely to turn to serious leisure to ride out the dispiriting effects of their economic plight. Lower-level employees are more often overwhelmed by being thrown out of work, suffering from depression and lethargy to an extent that leisure becomes next to impossible.[3] Part of the problem is that they feel useless and pressured by social convention to continually search for work, a frame of mind that alienates them from true leisure. In short, they are too demoralized to engage in leisure, which is useful activity designed to achieve a particular end. Meanwhile, sitting around bored to tears is no more leisure than it is work.

Moreover, Reid and Mannell and Aronowitz and DiFazio have found that, although workers aspire to more time after work and more leisure, they fail to see leisure playing a central role in their lives, even in retirement. This attitude toward work and leisure holds despite the increasingly routine, unattractive character of most work these days. For many people the appeal of modern work is largely external, offering mainly a paycheck and social connections.

Is a World of Leisure Possible?

Still, ever-growing numbers of workers have no choice in the matter: electronic technology is forcing them out of full-time employment and, increasingly, out of gainful employment of any kind. As a consequence, after-work time is growing at the expense of in-work time and, whatever your evaluation of work with respect to leisure, you will likely soon be in a position to experience much more leisure and much less work. My aim in this book has been to show you that worthwhile, dignified, serious leisure exists and that, whether it is pursued as a replacement for or a supplement to work, it can serve as a powerful central life interest with an appealing identity and lifestyle of its own.

One major legacy of the electronic revolution is the challenge of making the pursuit of serious leisure possible for large segments of the population. A number of thinkers have risen to this challenge and proposed solutions, several of which are presented below. In discussing them, I am assuming that once a person is effectively retired, that is, he or she is no longer searching for work, being unemployed is much less threatening and serious leisure is more favorably regarded as an activity in its own right. Research by Aronowitz and DiFazio suggests this assumption is justified:

> Recipients of guaranteed annual income who are relieved of most obligations to engage in labor do not fall apart. The incidence of alcoholism, divorce, and other social ills associated with conditions of dysfunctionality does not increase among men who are not working. Nor do they tend to experience higher rates of mortality than those of comparable age who are engaged in full-time work. Given the opportunity to engage in active nonwork [i.e., serious leisure], they choose this option virtually every time.[4]

Can any society afford to let a sizeable segment of its population devote itself to non-paid amateur, hobbyist and career volunteer pursuits in lieu of working at paid jobs, accepting for the sake of argument the assumption that jobs will be available on the same scale as in the past?

Several proposals are presented in the following section, proposals subjected to more public discussion with each passing year. I don't intend to present an exhaustive list of the ways to meet the challenge. I simply want to illustrate how the challenge might be met and that the route to widespread serious leisure is a possibility. These proposals are controversial, in part because each suffers from certain weaknesses, in part because each runs counter to the prevailing ideology of work. To be sure, some of them may seem unrealistic in the present and some may prove to be unrealistic in the future, yet strategies like establishing a minimum wage and restricting overtime employment have already been tried in Europe with a significant degree of success. Since a discussion of their controversial aspects would take us too far afield, readers interested in them are encouraged to turn to the works of Schor, Rifkin, Aronowitz and DiFazio, where they are considered in somewhat greater detail (see Works Cited).

Meeting the Challenge

Several thinkers have developed elaborate proposals describing how industrial society can survive, if not flourish, with fewer person-hours of work and more person-hours of leisure. Juliet Schor suggests that we substantially reduce our need for money and paid employment by either reducing the quantity of goods and services we consume or changing the ways we consume them or, preferably, living according to both principles. Her proposal closely resembles the consumer attitude espoused by the voluntary simplicity movement. For example, the latter urges believers to lower their overall personal consumption by purchasing fewer things and avoiding fads, as well as buying products known to be durable, energy efficient and easy to repair. It further urges them to walk, car-pool, ride bicycles and take public transit. Finally, this movement encourages membership in consumer- and worker-owned cooperatives, since these organizations can often supply goods and services more cheaply than their counterparts in the private sector.[5]

Schor shares with the voluntary simplicity movement the idea of buying only what we need to realize our occupational and serious leisure goals, while eschewing conspicuous, fad-driven consumption. People who follow her suggestions may discover they have also reduced their need to work a second job or even maintain a dual family income. The result: more free time becomes available for those who choose simplicity and more jobs become available for those who must work to finance goals that harmonize with voluntary simplicity.

Schor and the proponents of simple living show how people can pursue their goals using the reduced income most of them will be forced to accept in the future. Other proposals tackle the problem from a different angle, suggesting ways to provide for people whose income from work is insufficient. Each requires government intervention for its implementation, whether through legislation and/or payments to qualifying individuals.

RESTRICT EXTRA WORK One way to provide income in a society where there isn't enough work to go around is to limit by law the number of job-hours any one person can work. Accordingly, there are proposals for restricting or eliminating moonlighting, holding second jobs and working overtime. For example, discussions have been held in both Canada and the United States on the feasibility of a regulation that would force the larger employers to pay excessively high rates for overtime to check their use of it. At present, although they must pay higher wages for overtime than for work done during regular hours, overtime rates are still more economical than hiring new employees. The cost of fringe benefits for new employees is the principal saving when overtime is used.

Reducing the number of dual-income families by forcing them to become single-income families could open up an enormous number of jobs for the unemployed. Maureen Moore reported in 1989 that over 61% of all Canadian families had two incomes, usually with the wife and husband serving as co-heads of the household. A similar proportion has been observed in the United States.[6] Yet Christopher Sarlo notes in his book entitled *Poverty in Canada* that, although this trend is due in part to the desire of the both adults in the household to work, pure materialism also plays a prominent role. A significant proportion of dual-income families need the second wage, not to survive, but to keep up with the Joneses. To my knowledge, this proposal has never been tried, which is hardly surprising given the uproar it would cause when many families are struggling financially.

OFFER SHADOW WAGES Rifkin proposes that governments issue tax deduction vouchers to volunteers, calculated on the basis of the number of hours of service given to legally-certified, tax-exempt organizations. The deductions would constitute a "shadow wage" earned by underemployed workers. This wage would offset, in proportion to the number of hours of volunteering, the taxes owed by these volunteers, whether personal or property taxes. As an alternative, the vouchers could be used to obtain government goods and services, an arrangement Kouri believes would be especially popular with the elderly:

For example, citizens could do volunteer jobs in agencies and earn units of service from government agencies of their choice. They could exchange their vouchers for such items as tickets to municipal opera performances or tuition at a community college where they could study new skills to use in paid jobs.[7]

This proposal brings to the fore the Third Sector and the prominent role it is destined to play in the Information Age. This sector is the non-profit, voluntary action part of the economy; it stands apart from the sectors of government and for-profit, private industry. The Third Sector encompasses charitable organizations and philanthropic foundations, as well as the world of informal helping. Because goods and services are provided here, this sector is estimated to generate billions of dollars in economic value. Rifkin, Aronowitz and DiFazio, among others, see a greatly expanded place for the Third Sector in the present and future where government response to diminished revenues is, and will continue to be, to cut or reduce many publicly-funded health, social and educational programs and services.

While there will be some demand for casual volunteering in the expanded Third Sector, most volunteering will be of the serious, career variety. Nevertheless, it will only be career volunteering if it is defined by the volunteers as leisure rather than another obligated activity. In other words, if volunteer work leading to tax deductions is to become a genuine part of your optimal leisure lifestyle, you must feel free to abandon it if it becomes unsatisfying. The career volunteer should not be dependent on the shadow wages earned, should feel no obligation to work for them.

OFFER SOCIAL WAGES These same criteria of choice and satisfaction should also be applied to Rifkin's proposal for "social wages." This is government money given to the unemployed for the volunteer work they do, in effect the same money they received as welfare payments in more affluent times. Some of today's unemployed can be trained to work in complicated Third Sector roles. But again, since they are dependent on the income they receive, it is illogical to argue that these "volunteers" are pursuing serious leisure. Even though some will find satisfaction in these roles, they are still obligated to fill them, just as they were with the paying jobs.

Many workers receiving social wages will work side by side with true, unpaid volunteers, creating problems for their managers that they and researchers in the social sciences have only begun to confront. After studying volunteers in seven different organizations, all of which were also managed by volunteers, Jone Pearce concluded that

> the tension that can exist between volunteer and employee co-workers remains one of the unpleasant secrets of nonprofit organizations. The preceding discussion described how volunteers and employees, by the very nature of their different relationships to the organization, tend to undermine each other's legitimacy. Employees have higher professional and expertise-based status while undermining the legitimacy of volunteer "sacrifice" by taking salaries for their work. Volunteers give of themselves to the organization, yet undermine the professionalism of employees.[8]

Still, Pearce found that damaging levels of volunteer-employee conflict developed in only one of the organizations she investigated.

OFFER A GUARANTEED MINIMUM INCOME People unable to earn enough money through gainful employment, shadow wages or social wages, would be protected from poverty by a government-sponsored guaranteed minimum income program. In other words, government would catch these people in its social safety net, to provide reasonable food, clothing, shelter and other necessities of life. Rifkin concludes that such programs as do exist have met with varying degrees of success. Aronowitz and DiFazio hold that a program of this nature has never been tried in the United States because of the

> fiction that ours is a full-employment economy and joblessness is a temporary condition. . . . Beyond the obvious market assumption that keeping jobless benefits low encourages workers to reenter the paid labor force, all of these programs are suffused with a Christian moralism that regards the long-term poor as essentially irresponsible.[9]

In spite of the many obstacles, this proposal for meeting the challenge clearly offers the widest scope for pursuing serious leisure of any in this chapter. People assured a minimum income would literally be paid so they could play, "play" being synonymous with leisure. Most of the supporters of guaranteed minimal income plans have in mind more fulfilling and deeply satisfying activities for the recipients than casual leisure. Furthermore, these supporters envision that most of the people who would benefit from these plans would be at least middle-aged and made redundant or taken early retirement.

Where their pensions are inadequate, these former workers would turn to government payments to close the gap between poverty and an economic lifestyle enabling them to pursue one or two of the less expensive forms of serious leisure. At this level a number of serious leisure activities are plainly out of reach. But the recipients of a minimum income can participate in the many substantial activities demanding little or no cash outlay, among them chess, bridge, reading (library books), theater, bird-watching and archaeology as well as a great variety of career volunteer activities. Thus conceived and implemented, guaranteed minimum income plans would make it possible for the less well-to-do members of society to also experience Aristotle's maxim that the end of work is leisure.

OFFER HIGHER WAGES Some economists are proposing, as an alternative to shadow wages, that part-time workers be paid a higher wage for the smaller amount of work they do. This adjustment, in effect, would make their income equal to that of a full-time employee with the same experience filling the same role. Whereas few workers would oppose this solution to the challenge of the Information Age and its jobless future, many owners and managers of businesses would. After all, saving money by cutting employment costs has been the dominant motive and strategy behind the dramatic reduction in job opportunities we are now witnessing. From their point of view, paying a worker the same wage for performing less work is just plain ludicrous. Indeed, the present tendency is to try to squeeze more work from each employee for the same wage or, in many industries, for a reduced wage.

Nevertheless, some employers realize that granting certain personal advantages to their employees can pay off handsomely in worker loyalty and contentment. Thus a 25- or 30-hour work week can add badly needed flexibility to the hectic daily round of a dual-income family. Moreover, a shorter work week can enable some employees to pursue a serious leisure activity accompanied by a rise in personal well-being. It is possible, too, that workers receiving the same paycheck for 25 hours of work they once received for 40 hours of work will feel less exploited by their employers and will be more disposed to do their best for them in return.

The Leisure Age

One inevitable outcome of the first four proposals will be that the ordinary citizen will have much less money in pocket than before. That means less money for the necessities of life and less for leisure, whether casual or serious. The trade-off for people is that they will now have substantially more time after work to pursue activities of their choice, some of which – the serious ones – can provide tremendous returns in the form of profound satisfaction, attractive lifestyles and distinctive personal identities.

Thus, quite apart from the benefits it is now producing – notably for big business, big government and the knowledge sector – the Information Age holds the potential for giving birth to the Leisure Age. Modern society might act as midwife in assisting the arrival of this new epoch. Nonetheless, we must implement the proposals as soon as possible, before a large proportion of the population is socially and psychologically destroyed by the revolutionary changes afoot.

Bruce O'Hara, author of *Working Harder isn't Working*, argues that the next move lies with ordinary people. They must organize coalitions of labor, environmental, anti-poverty and pro-family groups and then try to redirect the attention of their members toward meeting the challenge. Our political leaders are in a dilemma about the long-term effects of the Information Age; they have little or no idea what to do next. Yet, although perplexed, they are open to suggestions. The corporate elite, when not obsessed with immediate financial gain, are as baffled. Yet according to Hugh Menzies, the more visionary of these are now aware that they are going to have contribute from their own extraordinary profits of today to help meet the challenge of tomorrow.[10]

In short, says O'Hara, ordinary people must speak up so they can be heard by those who make the decisions in modern society. People must seize the initiative and begin to direct social and economic change that can foster serious leisure. At the moment, the tendency among many leaders of industrialized states is to try to return to the past. Consequently, a stultifying conservative and even ultraconservative pall hangs over the contemporary politico-economic scene, the most immediate effects of which include repressing imaginative and fruitful solutions to the challenge, accompanied by unnecessarily heavy human social and psychological loss.

Perhaps the best way to make the point that a future with no work for some and only part-time work for many others is a good thing is for people to take up a serious leisure pursuit and experience first-hand the profound social and personal benefits it can give. Direct experience is a most effective antidote to ignorance born of a lack of participation. With such experience, people will be in a position to trumpet the virtues of a truly satisfying after-work lifestyle that can offer a leisure identity at least as distinctive and absorbing as the work identity that once dominated as the central life interest of Western civilization.

Endnotes

[1] Reid and Mannell, "The Globalization of the Economy and Potential New Roles for Work and Leisure."

[2] Haworth, "Meaningful Activity and Psychological Models of Non-employed."

[3] Kay, "Active Unemployment."

[4] Aronowitz and DiFazio, *The Jobless Future*, p. 336.

[5] Elgin, *Voluntary Simplicity*, pp. 34-36.

[6] Moore, "Dual-Earner Families"; U.S. Bureau of the Census, *Statistical Abstract of the United States*, Table 737.

[7] Kouri, *Volunteerism and Older Adults*, p. 14.

[8] Pearce, *Volunteers*, pp. 177-178.

[9] Aronowitz and DiFazio, *The Jobless Future*, p. 320.

[10] Hugh Menzies, "Who'll Plug the Safety-Net Hole?"

A Practical Bibliography of Serious Leisure

This bibliography contains many of the most recent books that describe particular amateur and hobbyist activities and set out ways to make contact with other participants and get started. There is also a short section of books on career volunteering in general. The books are listed according to activity in the same order as through the rest of the book. The most recent books are listed first. Readers who would like to find more books on their chosen activity can do so in any good-sized library or bookstore or in the Amazon Books Web site at http://www.amazon.com (use the subject search engine to explore its 2.5 million titles).

Although books provide the most extensive discussion of a given activity, its social world includes certain major events, organizations and periodicals about which you might want to know more. I have accumulated some information on a number of these, that I am most willing to share. I can be reached by mail at the Department of Sociology, University of Calgary, Calgary, Alberta, Canada, T2N 1N4; by telephone at (403) 220-5827; or by e-mail at stebbins@acs.ucalgary.ca. Please be sure to indicate your serious leisure interests.

Fine Arts - Music

Jazz

Scott D. Reeves, *Creative Beginnings: An Introduction to Jazz Improvisation* (Prentice-Hall, 1996).

Scott D. Reeves, *Creative Jazz Improvisation*, 2nd ed. (Prentice-Hall, 1995).

Stephen M. Stroff, *Discovering Great Jazz: A New Listener's Guide to the Sounds and Styles of Top Musicians and Their Recordings on CDs, Lps, and Cassettes* (Newmarket Press, 1991).

Choral *(see also Entertainment – Musical Theater)*

Susan Sutherland, *Singing* (Teach Yourself Books, 1995).

Ronald Combs and Robert Bowker, *Learning to Sing Nonclassical Music* (Prentice-Hall, 1994).

Jan Schmidt, *Basics of Singing*, 3rd ed. (Schirmer Books, 1993).

Operatic *(see also Fine Arts – Music [Choral])*

Barrymore Laurence Scherer, *Bravo: A Guide to the Opera for the Perplexed* (E.P. Dutton, 1996).

Mary Hamilton, *A-Z of Opera* (Facts on File, 1990).

Chamber Music

James Christensen, *Chamber Music: Notes for Players* (Distinctive, 1992).

Lester Chafetz, *The Ill Tempered String Quartet: A Vademecum for the Amateur Musician* (McFarland, 1989).

Orchestral

Robert R. Craven (ed.), *Symphony Orchestras of the World: Selected Profiles* (Greenwood, 1987).

Herbert Chappell, *Sounds Magnificent: The Story of the Symphony* (Parkwest, 1986).

Robert R. Craven (ed.), *Symphony Orchestras of the United States: Selected Profiles* (Greenwood, 1986).

Fine Arts – Dance

Ballet

Kate Castle, *Ballet* (Kingfisher Books, 1996).

Susan Au, *Ballet and Modern Dance* (Thames & Hudson, 1988).

Oleg Briansky and Vera S. Kostrovitskaya, *100 Lessons in Classical Ballet* (Proscenium, 1987).

Contemporary Dance

Susan Au, *Ballet and Modern Dance* (Thames & Hudson, 1988).

Fine Arts – Theatre

Community Theater

Jack Cassin-Scott, *Amateur Dramatics* (Cassell Academic, 1992).

Richard Boleskavski, *Acting: The First Six Lessons* (Theatre Art Books, 1987).

Edwin C. White, *Acting and Stage Movements* (Meriwether, 1985).

Robert A. Stebbins, *Amateurs: On the Margin between Work and Leisure* (Sage, 1979).

Robert E. Gard and Gertrude S. Burley, *Community Theatre* (Greenwood, 1975).

Dennis Castle, *Beginner's Guide to Amateur Acting* (Transatlantic Arts, 1973).

Pantomime

Tony Montanaro and Karen Hurll Montanaro, *Mime Spoken Here: The Performer's Portable Workshop* (Tilbury House, 1995).

Stefan Niedzialkowski and Jonathan Winslow, *Beyond the Word: The World of Mime* (Momentum Books, 1993).

Claude Kipnis, *The Mime Book*, 2nd ed. (Meriwether, 1990).

Cindie Straub and Matthew Straub, *Mime: Basics for Beginners* (Plays, 1984).

Art-Cinematic

Preston Blair, *Cartoon Animation* (Walter Foster, 1995).

Steven Bernstein, *Film Production* (Focal Press, 1994).

Jerry Bloedow, *Filmmaking Foundations* (Focal Press, 1991).

Kit Laybourne, *The Animation Book* (Crown, 1979).

Experimental

Margaret Croyden, *Lunatics, Lovers, and Poets: The Contemporary Experimental Theater* (McGraw-Hill, 1974).

Fine Arts – Art

Painting

Miranda Fellows, *100 Keys to Great Watercolor Painting* (North Light Books, 1994).

Stephen Quiller, *Acrylic Painting Techniques / How to Master the Medium of Our Age* (Watson-Guptill Publications, 1994).

Adrian Hill, *Adrian Hill's Oil Painting for Beginners* (Sterling, 1994).

Photography

George Schaub, *The Art & Craft of Black & White Photography* (NTC, 1996).

Aaron Scharf, *Art and Photography* (Penguin USA, 1995).

Brian F. Peterson, *Learning to See Creatively* (Amphoto, 1988).

Bill Smith, *Designing a Photograph: Creative Techniques for Making Your Photographs Work* (Watson-Guptill, 1986).

Drawing

Clint Brown and Cheryl McLean, *Drawing from Life* (Harcourt Brace Jovanovich, 1992).

Burne Hogarth, *Dynamic Drawing* (Watson-Guptill, 1990).

Printing

Judy Kastin, *100 Keys to Great Calligraphy* (North Light Books, 1996).

David Harris, *The Art of Calligraphy* (Dorling-Kindersley, 1995).

Judy Martin and Miriam Stribley, spiral ed. *Calligraphy Skills and Techniques* (Macmillan, 1994).

Printmaking

Bernard Toale, *Basic Printmaking Techniques* (Davis, 1992).

Anthony Griffiths, *Prints and Printmaking: An Introduction to the History and Techniques* (University of California Press, 1996).

Walter Koschatzky, *Art of the Print: History, Technique, Master Works* (Abaris Books, 1996).

Sculpting and Ceramics

Susan Peterson, *The Craft and Art of Clay*, 2nd ed. (Prentice-Hall, 1996).

Paul Jackson, *The Art and Craft of Paper Sculpture* (Chilton, 1996).

David Swinton, *The Magic of Paper Sculpture* (Cassell Academic, 1996).

Leon I. Nigrosh, *Claywork: Form and Idea in Ceramic Design*, 3rd ed. (Sterling, 1994).

Nathan C. Hale, *Creating Welded Sculpture* (Dover, 1994).

Joseph Amendola, *Ice Carving Made Easy*, 2nd ed. (Van Nostrand Reinhold, 1994).

Fine Arts – Literature
Fiction

Ann Copeland, *The ABC's of Writing Fiction* (Story Press, 1996).

Nancy Kress, *Beginnings, Middles, and Ends (The Elements of Fiction Writing)* (Writers Digest Books, 1993).

Barnaby Conrad, *The Complete Guide to Writing Fiction* (Writers Digest Books, 1990).

Orson S. Card, *Characters and Viewpoints (The Elements of Fiction Writing)* (Writers Digest Books, 1988).

Poetry

Paul Agostino, *Creative Writing: Poetry from New Angles* (Prentice-Hall, 1996).

M. Ryan, *How to Read and Write Poems* (Franklin Watts, 1991).

Myra Cohn Livingston, *Poem-Making: Ways to Begin Writing Poetry* (HarperCollins, 1991).

Non-fiction

Lee Gutkind, *The Art of Creative Writing: Writing and Selling the Literature of Reality* (Wiley, 1997).

Philip Gerard, *Creative Nonfiction: Researching and Crafting Stories of Real Life* (Story Press, 1996).

Sophy Burnham, *For Writers Only* (on the pains and joys of writing) (Ballantine Books, 1994).

Guide for Authors (Basil Blackwell, 1991).

Entertainment – Music
Folk and Country Music

Michael Stepaniak and Joanne Stepaniak, *Folk & Traditional Music Festivals: 1996 Guide for U.S. and Canada* (Shoreline, 1995).

Carl Sandburg, *The American Songbag* (Harcourt Brace, 1990).

Larry Sundberg and Dick Weissman, *The Folk Music Sourcebook* (Da Capo Press, 1989).

Rock

Del Hopkins and Margaret Hopkins, *Careers as a Rock Musician* (Rosen, 1993).

Charles T. Brown, *The Art of Rock and Roll*, 3rd ed. (Prentice-Hall, 1992).

Richard Meltzer, *The Aesthetics of Rock* (Da Capo Press, 1988).

Entertainment – Dance

Ballroom

Judy Patterson Wright, *Social Dance Instruction: Steps to Success* (Human Kinetics Publishing, 1995).

Walter Laird, *Ballroom Dance Pack: Book with CD/Step Cards/Feet Templates* (Dorling-Kindersley, 1994).

Barbara Early, *Finding the Best Dance Instruction* (Betterway, 1992).

Sally Sommer, Ken Graves and Eva Lipman, *Ballroom* (Milkweed Editions, 1989).

Country and Western

Jane A. Harris, Anne M. Pittman and Marlys S. Waller, *Dance a While: Handbook for Folk, Square, Contra, and Social Dance*, 7th ed. (Macmillan, 1994).

Myrna Martin Schild, *Square Dancing Everyone* (Hunter Textbooks, 1987).

Ronald Smedley, *Let's Dance – Country Style: A Handbook of Simple Traditional Dances*, rev. ed. (Wm. Collins & Sons, 1981).

Line Dancing

Christy Lane, *Christy Lane's Complete Book of Line Dancing* (Human Kinetics, 1994).

Ollie Mae Ray, *Encyclopedia of Line Dances* (American Alliance for Health Physical Education and Recreation, 1992).

Jazz Dance

Minda Goodman Kraines and Esther Pryor, *Jazz Dance: A Primer for the Beginning Jazz Dance Student* (Mayfield, 1996).

Lorraine Person Kriegel and Kimberly Chandler-Vaccaro, *Jazz Dance Today* (West, 1994).

Marshall W. Stearns, *Jazz Dance: The Story of American Vernacular Dance* (Da Capo Press, 1994).

Tap Dance

Anita Feldman, *Inside Tap: Technique and Improvisation for Today's Tap Dancer* (Princeton Book, 1996).

Roy Castle, *Roy Castle on Tap: His Unique Tap Dancing Course* (David & Charles, 1987).

Entertainment – Theatre

Public Speaking

Rudolph F. Verderber, *The Challenge of Effective Speaking*, 10th ed. (Wadsworth, 1996).

John Hasling, *The Audience, the Message, the Speaker*, 5th ed. (McGraw-Hill, 1992).

Page Emory Moyer, *The ABC's of a Really Good Speech* (Circle Press, 1990).

Magic

Guy Frederick and Jason Hurst, *101 Classic Magic Tricks* (Sterling, 1995).

Robert A. Stebbins, *Career, Culture, and Social Psychology in a Variety Art: The Magician* (Krieger, 1993).

Bill Severn and Timothy Wenk, *Bill Severn's Amazing Magic* (Stackpole Books, 1992).

Henry Hay, *The Amateur Magician's Handbook*, 4th ed. (New American Library, 1983).

Stand-Up Comedy

Gene Perret, *Successful Stand-Up Comedy* (Samuel French, 1994).

Sharon Menzel-Gerrie, *Careers in Comedy* (Rosen, 1993).

Robert A. Stebbins, *The Laugh-Makers: Stand-Up Comedy as Art, Business, and Lifestyle* (McGill-Queen's University Press, 1990).

Judy Carter, *Stand-Up Comedy* (Dell Books, 1989).

Variety Arts (Puppetry, Clowning, Juggling, Ventriloquism)

Kolby King, *Ventriloquism Made Easy* (Dover, 1997).

Catherine Perkins, *The Most Excellent Book on How to Be a Clown* (Copper Beech Books, 1996).

Ivan Bulloch and Diane James, *A Juggler (I want to Be)* (World Book, 1995).

Bobby Besmehn, *Juggling Step-by-Step* (Sterling, 1995).

Bruce Fife, Tony Blanco and Steve Kissell, *Creative Clowning*, 2nd ed. (Piccadilly Books, 1992).

Bruce Taylor, *Marionette Magic: From Concept to Curtain Call* (Tab Books, 1989).

Edgar Bergen, *How to Become a Ventriloquist* (Amereon, 1988).

Happy Jack Feder, *The Independent Entertainer: How to Be a Successful Clown, Mime, Magician, or Puppeteer* (Prentice-Hall, 1982).

Musical Theater (see also Fine Arts – Music [Choral])

Richard Kislan, *The Musical: A Look at the American Musical Theater* (Applause Theatre Book, 1995).

David Craig, *On Singing Onstage* (Applause Theatre Book, 1991).

Michael Bawtree, *New Singing Theatre: A Charter for the Music Theatre Movement* (Oxford University Press, 1991).

Entertainment – Art

The basic techniques of the commercial arts are generally the same as those of the equivalent fine arts. Nevertheless, additional information exists in some entertainment fields.

Drawing

Renzo Barto, *How to Draw Cartoon Characters* (Troll Associates, 1994).

Sculpture

Captain Visual, *Captain Visual's Big Book of Balloon Art: A Complete Book of Balloonology for Beginners and Advanced Twisters* (Citadel Press, 1995).

Bruce Fife, *Balloon Sculpting: A Fun and Easy Guide to Making Balloon Animals, Toys, and Games* (Empire, 1994).

Woodcarving

Ian Norbury, *Projects for Creative Woodcarving* (Linden, 1996).

Antony Denning, *The Art and Craft of Woodcarving: A Complete Course with Twelve Original Projects* (Running Press, 1994).

Elmer J. Tangerman, *Complete Guide to Woodcarving* (Sterling, 1984).

Sports

The team sports are not covered on this Bibliography, since people normally fall in love with them by watching others play and learning the rudiments through observation. The beginner's next step, depending on the sport, is to join a team or take lessons. Either way, he or she learns the basic techniques. Entry into the individual sports is different, however. Self-instruction is possible, and books have been written on the basic techniques of many of them.

Individual sports (professional)

Tennis

Julie Jensen, *Beginning Tennis* (Lerner, 1995).

Marc Miller and Andy King, *Fundamental Tennis* (Lerner, 1995).

Paul Douglas, *Handbook of Tennis*, rev. ed. (Knopf, 1992).

Golf

Thomas D. Fahey, *Basic Golf* (Mayfield, 1995).

John A. May, *Complete Book of Golf: A Guide to Equipment, Techniques, and Courses* (Gallery Books, 1994).

Larry Dennis, *A Beginner's Guide to Golf* (National Golf Foundation, 1993).

Squash and Racquetball

Pippa Sales, *Improve Your Squash Game: 101 Drills, Coaching Tips, and Resources* (Disa, 1996).

Woody Clouse, Ed Turner and Edward T. Turner, *Winning Racquetball: Skills, Drills, and Strategies* (Human Kinetics, 1995).

Jahangir Khan, Keven Pratt and Matthew Ward, *Learn Squash and Racquetball in a Weekend* (Knopf, 1993).

Eric Sommers, *Squash: Technique, Tactics, Training* (Crowood Press, 1992).

Stan Kittleson, *Racquetball: Steps to Success* (Leisure Press, 1991).

Equestrian

J.P. Forget, *The Complete Guide to Western Horsemanship* (Howell Book House, 1995).

Eleanor F. Prince and Gaydell M. Collier, *Basic Horsemanship: English and Western*, rev. ed. (Doubleday, 1993).

Brenda Imus, *From the Ground Up: Horsemanship for the Adult Rider* (Howell Book House, 1992).

Bowling

Robert H. Strickland, *Bowling: Steps to Success*, 2nd ed. (Human Kinetics, 1996).

Doug Werner, *Bowler's Start-Up: A Beginner's Guide to Bowling*, spiral ed. (Tracks, 1995).

Carol Blassingame and Thomas S. Cross, *Success in Bowling Through Practical Fundamentals* (Kendall Hunt, 1991).

Figure Skating

Margaret Blackstone and Toni Goffe, *This is Figure Skating* (Henry Holt, 1997).

Patricia Hagen (ed.), *Figure Skating: Sharpen Your Skills* (Masters Press, 1995).

Motorcycle Racing

Jeff Savage, *Motocross Cycles* (Capstone Press, 1996).

Jeremy Evans, *Motocross & Trials* (Crestwood House, 1994).

Michael Dregni, *Motorcycle Racing* (Capstone Press, 1994).

Individual Sports (elite amateur)

Handball

Richard C. Nelson and Harlan S. Berger, *Handball* (Prentice-Hall, 1971).

B.J. Rowland, *Handball: A Complete Guide* (Transatlantic Arts, 1970).

Swimming

Jane Katz, *The Aquatic Handbook for Lifetime Fitness* (Allyn & Bacon, 1996).

Steve Tarpinian, *The Essential Swimmer* (Lyons & Burford, 1996).

Phillip Whitten and Ethan Berry, *The Complete Book of Swimming* (Random House, 1994).

Track and Field

Steve Boga, *Runners and Walkers: Keeping Pace with the World's Best* (Stackpole Books, 1993).

Gerry A. Carr, *Fundamentals of Track and Field* (Leisure Press, 1991).

Gary Wright, *Track and Field: A Step-By-Step Guide* (Troll Associates, 1991).

Archery

John Adams, *Archery* (Stackpole Books, 1996).

Kathleen Haywood and Catherine F. Lewis, *Archery: Steps to Success*, 2nd ed. (Leisure Press, 1996).

Roger Combs, *Archer's Digest*, 6th ed. (DBI Books, 1995).

Badminton

Tony Grice, *Badminton: Steps to Success* (Human Kinetics, 1996).

Steve Boga, *Badminton* (Stackpole Books, 1996).

Martial Arts

Steve Potts, *Mastering Martial Arts* (Capstone Press, 1996).

Michael Maliszewski, *Spiritual Dimensions of the Martial Arts* (Charles E. Tuttle, 1996).

Ron Sieh and Terry Wilson, *Martial Arts for Beginners* (Writers & Readers, 1995).

Speed Skating

Dianne Holum, *Complete Handbook of Speed Skating* (Enslow, 1984).

Richard Arnold, *Better Sport Skating* (David & Charles, 1983).

Alpine Skiing and Snowboarding

Jeff Bennett and Scott Downey, *The Complete Snowboarder* (McGraw-Hill, 1994).

Carol Poster and Lucie Lavallee, *The Basic Essentials of Alpine Skiing* (Ice Books, 1993).

John Yacenda, *Alpine Skiing: Steps to Success* (Leisure Press, 1992).

Paul McCallum and Christine L. McCallum, *The Downhill Skiing Handbook* (Betterway, 1992).

John McMullen, *The Basic Essentials of Snowboarding* (Ice Books, 1991).

Cross-Country Skiing

Sindre Bergen and Bob O'Connor, *Cross-Country Skiing* (Masters Press, 1997).

Brian Cazeneuve, *Cross-Country Skiing: A Complete Guide* (W.W. Norton, 1995).

John Moynier and Li Newton, *The Basis Essentials of Cross-Country Skiing* (Ice Books, 1990).

Cycling

Peter Oliver, *Bicycling: Trail and Touring Basics* (W.W. Norton, 1996).

Jeremy Evans, *Cycling on Road and Trail* (Crowood Press, 1996).

Eugene A. Sloane, *The Complete Book of Bicycling*, 4th ed. (Fireside, 1988).

Shooting (firearms)

John Malloy, *Complete Guide to Guns & Shooting* (DBI Books, 1995).

Stepheni Slahor, *Beginner's Shooting Guide: With Some Tips from Experts* (Allegheny Press, 1986).

Gymnastics

Don Gutman, *Gymnastics* (Viking Press, 1996).

Paul Joseph, *Gymnastics* (Adbo & Daughters, 1996).

Julie Jensen and Andy King, *Beginning Gymnastics* (Lerner, 1995).

Wrestling

Jeff Savage, *Wrestling Basics* (Capstone Press, 1996).

William A. Martell, *Greco-Roman Wrestling* (Human Kinetics, 1993).

Robert Sandelson, *Combat Sports (Olympic Sports)* (Crestwood House, 1991).

Fencing

Nick Evangelista, *The Art and Science of Fencing* (Masters Press, 1996).

Charles Simonian, *Basic Foil Fencing*, 4th ed. (Kendall Hunt, 1995).

Aldo Nadi, *On Fencing* (Laureate Press, 1994).

Canoe and Kayak Racing

Eric Evans, *Whitewater Racing* (Van Nostrand Reinhold, 1981).

Gordon Richards, *Complete Book of Canoeing and Kayaking* (Horizon Book Promotions, 1981).

Fred Heese, *Canoe Racing* (Contemporary Books, 1979).

Sailing

Stephen Colgate, *Fundamentals of Sailing, Cruising, and Racing*, rev. ed. (W.W. Norton, 1996).

David Seidman and Kelly Mulford, *The Complete Sailor: Learning the Art of Sailing* (International Marine, 1995).

M.B. George, *Basic Sailing* (William Morrow, 1984).

Science

Computer Science

Larry Long and Nancy Long, *Introduction to Computers & Information Systems: The Internet Edition*, 5th ed. (Prentice-Hall, 1996).

M. Morris Mano and Charles R. Kime, *Logic and Computer Design Fundamentals* (Prentice-Hall, 1996).

Rick Decker and Stuart Hirschfield, *The Analytical Engine: An Introduction to Computer Science Using Hypercard 2.1* (with disk), 2nd ed. (PWS, 1994).

Astronomy

Robert A. Garfinkle, *Star-Hopping: Your Visa to Viewing the Universe* (Cambridge University Press, 1994).

Fred Schaaf, *The Amateur Astronomer: Explorations and Investigations* (Franklin Watts, 1994).

Chet Raymo, *365 Starry Nights: An Introduction to Astronomy for Every Night of the Year* (Simon & Schuster, 1992).

John B. Sidgwick, *Amateur Astronomer's Handbook* (Dover, 1980).

Mineralogy

George W. Robinson and Jeffery A. Scovil, *Minerals: An Illustrated Exploration of the Dynamic World of Minerals and Their Properties* (Simon & Schuster, 1994).

Andrew Putnis, *An Introduction to Mineral Sciences* (Cambridge University Press, 1992).

Lloyd H. Barrow, *Adventures with Rocks and Minerals* (Enslow, 1991).

Meteorology

H. Michael Mogil and Barbara G. Levine, *The Amateur Meteorologist: Explorations and Investigations* (Franklin Watts, 1993).

Richard A. Anthes, *Meteorology*, 7th ed. (Prentice-Hall, 1996).

Joseph M. Moran and Michael D. Moran, *Essentials of Weather* (Prentice-Hall, 1994).

Ornithology

Frank B. Gill, *Ornithology*, 2nd ed. (W.H. Freeman, 1994).

Lester L. Short, *The Lives of Birds: The Birds of the World and Their Behavior* (Henry Holt, 1993).

Colin Harrison and Howard Luxton, *The Bird: Master of Flight* (Barrons Educational Series, 1993).

Entomology

Christopher O'Toole, *Alien Empire: An Exploration of the Life of Insects* (HarperCollins, 1996).

Richard J. Elzinga, *Fundamentals of Entomology*, 4th ed. (Prentice-Hall, 1996).

H. Steven Dashefsky, *Entomology* (Tab Books, 1994).

Botany

Penny R. Durant and Nancy Woodman, *Exploring the World of Plants* (Franklin Watts, 1995).

Lorentz C. Peterson, *The Diversity and Evolution of Plants* (CRC Press, 1995).

Jorie Hunken, *Botany for All Ages: Discovering Nature through Activities for Children and Adults*, 2nd ed. (Globe Pequot Press, 1994).

History (general)

Mark T. Gilderhus, *History and Historians: A Historiographical Introduction* (Prentice-Hall, 1996).

Robert Skapura and John Marlowe, *History: A Student's Guide to Research and Writing* (Libraries Unlimited, 1988).

Marc Bloch, *Historian's Craft* (Random House, 1964).

History *(family)*

Jim Willard, Terry Willard and Jane Wilson, *Ancestors: A Beginner's Guide to Family History and Genealogy* (Houghton Mifflin, 1997).

Charley Kempthorne, *For All Time: A Complete Guide to Writing Your Family History* (Heinemann, 1996).

Archaeology

Brian M. Fagan, *Archaeology: A Brief Introduction*, 6th ed. (Longman, 1996).

Michael Avi-Yonah, *Dig This! How Archaeologists Uncover Our Past* (Runestone Press, 1993).

Bill McMillon, *The Archaeology Handbook: A Field Manual and Resource Guide* (John Wiley, 1991).

Robert A. Stebbins, *Amateurs: On the Margin between Work and Leisure* (Sage, 1979).

Collecting

Collecting *(general)*

no author given, *Garage Sale & Flea Market Annual*, 4th ed. (Collector Books, 1996).

Posters

Tony Fusco, *Posters: Identification and Price Guide*, 2nd ed. (Avon Books, 1994).

The 20th-Century Poster (Abbeville Press, 1990).

Coins, Currency and Medals

Scott A. Travers, *The Coin Collector's Survival Manual: An Indispensable Guide for Collectors and Investors*, 3rd ed. (Bonus Books, 1996).

Fred Schwan, *Collecting Coins* (National Book Network, 1996).

Scott A. Travers, *One-Minute Coin Expert*, 2nd ed. (House of Collectibles, 1996).

Collecting Medals and Decorations, 3rd ed. (Numismatic Fine Arts Intl., 1967).

Fred Schwan, *Collecting Paper Money* (National Book Network, 1996).

Barry Krause, *Collecting Paper Money for Pleasure & Profit A Comprehensive Guide and Handbook for Collectors and Investors* (Betterway, 1992).

Stamps

Neill Granger, *Stamp Collecting (First Guide)* (Millbrook Press, 1994).

Stanley M. Bierman, *Worlds Greatest Stamp Collectors* (Linns Stamp News, 1990).

Natural objects

Gerhard Lichter, *Fossil Collector's Handbook: Finding, Identifying, Preparing, Displaying* (Sterling, 1993).

Steve Parker and Raymond L. Bernor (editors), *The Practical Paleontologist* (Fireside, 1991).

Charles W. Chesterman, *National Audubon Society Field Guide to North American Rocks and Minerals* (Knopf, 1979).

S. Peter Dance, *The World's Shells: A Guide for Collectors* (McGraw-Hill, 1976).

Models

Ron Smith, *Collecting Toy Airplanes: An Identification & Value Guide* (Books Americana, 1995).

Richard O'Brien, *Collecting Toy Cars & Trucks (A Collector's Identification & Value Guide*, No. 1 (Books Americana, 1994).

John Grams, *Beginner's Guide to Toy Train Collecting and Operating*, Vol. 31 (Kalmbach, 1992).

Dolls

Dawn Herlocher, *200 Years of Dolls: Identification and Price Guide* (Antique Trader, 1996).

Kerry Taylor, *The Collector's Guide to Dolls: The Collectors Guide to Dolls (Collector's Guide Series)* (Smithmark, 1996).

Jane Foulke and Howard Foulke, *Insider's Guide to Doll Buying & Selling: Antique to Modern* (Hobby House Press, 1995).

Art objects (paintings)

Louisa Buck and Philip Dodd, *Relative Values: Or What's Art Worth?* (BBC, 1994).

Leonard Duboff, *The Art Business Encyclopedia* (Allworth Press, 1994).

Alan S. Bamberger, *Buy Art Smart* (Wallace-Homestead Book, 1990).

Art objects *(musical instruments)*

Robert Willcutt, *Musical Instrument Collector* (Bold Strummer, 1983).

Genevieve Dournon, *Guide for the Collection of Traditional Musical Instruments* (United Nations Educational, 1982).

Art objects *(figurines and plates)*

Robert L. Miller, *The No. 1 Price Guide to M. I. Hummel Figurines, Plates, More...*, 6th ed. (Bristol Books, 1995).

Margo Lewis and Herschell Gordon Lewis, *Everybody's Guide to Plate Collecting*, 2nd ed. (Bonus Books, 1994).

Carl F. Luckey, *Luckey's Hummel Figurines and Plates: A Collector's Identification and Value Guide*, 10th ed. (Books Americana, 1993).

Eleanor Clark, *Plate Collecting* (Lyle Stuart, 1980).

Antiques *(general)*

Ralph M. Kovel and Terry H. Kovel, *Kovels' Antiques & Collectibles Price List 1997*, 29th ed. (Crown, 1996).

Anthony Curtis, *The Lyle Official Antiques Review, 1997* (Perigee, 1996).

Don Bingham and Joan Bingham, *Buying and Selling Antiques and Collectibles: For Fun and Profit* (Charles E. Tuttle, 1994).

Antique Toys

Richard O'Brien, *Collecting Toys: A Collector's Identification & Value Guide*, 7th ed. (Books Americana, 1995).

Bob Huxford and Sharon Huxford (eds.), *Schroeder's Collectible Toys Antique to Modern Price Guide / 1996*, 2nd ed. (Collector Books, 1995).

David Longest, *Toys: Antique and Collectible* (Collector Books, 1990).

Antique Cars

Quentin Willson, *The Ultimate Classic Car Book*, 1st American ed. (Dorling-Kindersley, 1995).

John Gunnell (ed.), *Collector Car Digest: Old Cars* (Motorbooks International, 1993).

Beverly R. Kimes (ed.), *Classic Car: The Ultimate Book About the World's Grandest Automobiles* (Classic Car Club of America, 1990).

Antique Books

John Carter and Nicolas Barker, *ABC for Book Collectors*, 7th ed. (Lyons & Burford, 1995).

Estelle Ellis, Caroline Seebohm and Christopher S. Sykes, *At Home With Books: How Booklovers Live With and Care for Their Libraries* (Random House, 1995).

Edward N. Zempel and Linda A. Verkler (eds.), *Book Prices: Used and Rare, 1994* (Spoon River Press, 1994).

Antique Clocks, Watches and Bottles

Michael Polak, *Bottles: Identification and Price Guide* (Avon Books, 1994).

Alan Smith, *Clocks and Watches (Antique Collectors Guide)* (Crescent Books, 1989).

Antique Guns

Ian V. Hogg, *The Story of the Gun* (St. Martins Press, 1996).

John E. Traister, *Antique Guns: The Collector's Guide*, rev. ed. (Stoeger, 1994).

Joseph J. Schroeder (ed.), *Gun Collector's Digest*, 5th ed. (DBI Books, 1989).

Pop Culture (pins, cards, caps, comic books)

Deidre A. Sullivan, *Caps* (Andrews & McMeel, 1997).

Michael McKeever, *Instant Expert: Collecting Sports Cards* (National Book Network, 1996).

Thomas S. Owens, *Collecting Comic Books: A Young Person's Guide* (Millbrook Press, 1995).

Paula Spencer, *Olympic Games Countdown: The Official Book of Olympic Games Pin Collecting* (Coca Cola, 1994).

Sports Collectors Digest, *Getting Started in Card Collecting* (Krause, 1993).

Paul Green and Tony Galovich, *Collecting Baseball, Basketball, Football, Hockey Cards* (Bonus Books, 1992).

Making and Tinkering

Cooking, Baking and Candy-Making

Betty Crocker, *Betty Crocker's New Cookbook: Everything You Need to Know to Cook, 8th ed.* (MacMillan, 1996).

Norman Kolpas (ed.), *Dinner Parties* (HarperCollins, 1996).

Carole Bloom, *Truffles, Candies, & Confections: Elegant Candymaking in the Home,* 2nd ed. (Crossing Press, 1996).

Bick Malgieri and Tom Eckerle, *How to Bake: The Complete Guide to Perfect Cakes, Cookies, Pies, Tarts, Breads, Pizzas, Muffins, Sweet and Savory* (HarperCollins, 1995).

Joseph Amendola, *The Baker's Manual,* 4th ed. (Van Nostrand Reinhold, 1992).

Beverage Crafts

American Wine Society, *The American Wine Society Presents the Complete Handbook of Winemaking* (G. W. Kent, 1994).

R.M. Bryne, *How to Make Liqueurs* (Seven Hills Books, 1993).

Dave Miller, *Brewing the World's Great Beers: A Step-By-Step Guide* (HarperCollins, 1992).

Decorating activities

Amanda Pearce, Sally Burton, Stephen Butler and Gerry Copp, *The Crafter's Complete Guide to Collage* (Watson-Guptill, 1997).

Glenn McDean, *The Gilding Kit* (Watson-Guptill, 1996).

Juliet Bawden and Lucy Mason, *Mobile Magic: Innovative Ideas for Airborne Accessories* (Lorenz Books, 1996).

Mary MacCarthy, *Decorative Stencils for Your Home: An Imaginative Range of Stencils Inspired by the Arts & Crafts Movement* (North Light Books, 1996).

M. Masera and O. Rilke, *Dried Flowers: Stylish Arrangements to Decorate Your Home* (Ward Lock, 1996).

Holly Boswell, *The Decoupage Book: More Than 60 Decorative Projects Using Simple Techniques* (Lark Books, 1995).

Elizabeth Palmer, *Ikebana: The Art of Japanese Flower Arranging* (Book Sales, 1993).

Robert G. Bush, *Designs for Glass Etching* (Dover, 1989).

Interlacing and Interlocking Activities

Karen Elder and Christine Hanscomb, *Needlepoint* (Clarkson Potter, 1996).

Joyce E. Cusick, *Crafting with Lace: More than 40 Enchanting Projects to Make* (Lark Books, 1995).

Judith B. Montano, *Elegant Stitches: An Illustrated Stitch Guide and Source Book of Inspiration* (C & T, 1995).

Daisy Grubbs, *The Art and Craft of Quilting: A Beginner's Guide to Patchwork Design, Color, and Expression* (Watson-Guptill, 1995).

Pien Lemstra, *Baskets: Indoors Outdoors Practical Decorative* (Harry N. Abrams, 1995).

Deborah Chandler and Debbie Redding, *Learning to Weave*, rev. ed. (Interweave Press, 1995).

Nancy Harvey and Susan Harvey, *Tapestry Weaving: A Comprehensive Study Guide* (Interweave Press, 1991).

Alice Beatty and Mary Sargent, *Basic Rug Hooking*, 2nd ed. (Stackpole Books, 1990).

Maggie Righetti, *Crocheting in Plain English* (St. Martins Press, 1988).

Maggie Righetti, *Knitting in Plain English* (St. Martins Press, 1986).

Knot-making activities

John Van Vliet, *The Art of Fly Tying* (Cowles Creative, 1994).

Peter Owen, *The Book of Decorative Knots* (Lyons & Burford, 1994).

Toys (dollhouse furnishings)

Maurice Harper, *Make Your Own Dolls' House Furniture* (Sterling, 1995).

Vivienne Boulton, *The Dollhouse Decorator / The Complete Guide to Do-It-Yourself Furnishings for Dolls and Dollhouses* (Dorling-Kindersley, 1993).

Thelma R. Newman, *The Complete Book of Making Miniatures: For Room Settings and Dollhouses* (Crown, 1975).

Toy Puppets and Dolls

Argie Manolis (ed.), *The Doll Sourcebook* (Betterway, 1996).

Laura Ross, *Hand Puppets: How to Make and Use Them*, rev. ed. (Dover, 1990).

Toy Models

Mike Ashey, *Building 7 Detailing Scale Model Ships: The Complete Guide to Building, Detailing, Scratchbuilding, and Modifying Scale Model Ships* (Kalmbach, 1996).

Douglas R. Pratt, *Basics of Model Rocketry*, 2nd ed. (Kalmbach, 1996).

Harry G. Stine, *Handbook of Model Rocketry*, 6th ed. (John Wiley, 1994).

Keith Laumer, *How to Design and Build Flying Models*, rev. ed. (HarperCollins, 1970).

Toys and Games

Jeff Loader and Jennie Loader, *Making Wooden Toys & Games* (Sterling, 1995).

Paper crafts

Kathleen Ziegler and Nick Greco, *Paper Sculpture: A Step-By-Step Guide* (Rockport, 1996).

Rob Shepherd, *Hand-Made Books: An Introduction to Bookbinding* (Arthur Schwartz, 1995).

Peter Engel, *Origami from Angelfish to Zen* (Dover, 1994).

Lone Halse, *Papier Mache* (Parkwest, 1994).

Chris Rich, *The Book of Paper Cutting: A Complete Guide to All the Techniques – With More than 100 Project Ideas* (Lark Books, 1994).

Kathy Blake and Bill Milne, *Making & Decorating Your Own Paper: Innovative Techniques & Original Projects* (Sterling, 1994).

John Bringhurst, *Planes, Jets, & Helicopters: Great Paper Airplanes* (Tab Books, 1993).

Leather and Textile Activities

Singer Sewing Machine Company, *Sewing for the Home*, rev. ed. (Cowles Creative, 1996).

Gunilla P. Sjoberg, *Felt: New Directions for an Ancient Craft* (Interweave Press, 1996).

no author given, *The Complete Book of Sewing* (Dorling-Kindersley, 1996).

Kate Broughton, *Textile Dyeing: The Step-By-Step Guide and Showcase* (Rockport, 1996).

Valerie Michael, *The Leatherworking Handbook: A Practical Illustrated Sourcebook of Techniques and Projects* (Cassell Academic, 1995).

Reader's Digest, *Complete Guide to Sewing: Step-By-Step Techniques for Making Clothes*, rev. ed. (Readers's Digest, 1995).

Woodworking activities

Albert Jackson, David Day, Simon Jennings, *The Complete Manual of Woodworking* (Knopf, 1997).

Jim Tolpin, *Working Wood: A Complete Bench-Top Reference* (Davis, 1996).

David Hume, *Marquetry: How to Make Pictures and Patterns in Wood Veneers* (Arthur Schwartz, 1995).

Editors of Rodale Books, *The Weekend Woodworker: Projects for the Home Craftsman: Cabinets and Chests, Tables and Chairs, Kitchen Projects, Accents, Outdoor Projects, Toys* (Rodale Press, 1993).

Metalworking activities

Tim McCreight, *The Complete Metalsmith: An Illustrated Handbook*, rev. ed. (Davis, 1991).

Mike George, *Metalworking: A Manual of Techniques* (Crowood Press, 1991).

Do-It-Yourself Activities

Duffy, *Basic Car Care: Survival Guide* (Delmar, 1997).

Denise L. Caringer (ed.), *Additions: Your Guide to Planning and Remodeling* (Meredith Books, 1997).

Katie Hamilton and Gene Hamilton, *Do It Yourself...or Not?* (Berkley, 1996).

Michael Bishop and Dennis Holmes, *Tune-Up & Electrical Service: A Mini-Course for the Do-It-Yourselfer* (about cars) (Do It Right, 1994).

Better Homes and Gardens, *Better Homes and Gardens Complete Guide to Home Repair, Maintenance & Improvement* (Better Homes & Gardens Books, 1994).

Raising and Breeding Outdoor Plants

Cathy Hass, *Easy-Step Landscape Design* (Ortho Books, 1996).

Katie Hamilton and Gene Hamilton, *Gardening Made Easy* (Adams, 1996).

Better Homes and Gardens, *Better Homes and Gardens Lawns: The Gardener's Collection* (Better Homes & Gardens Books, 1995).

Janet H. Sanchez, *Lawns, Ground Covers & Vines* (Better Homes Gardens Books, 1995).

Peter Blackburne-Maze, *A Creative Step-By-Step Guide to Fruit and Vegetables* (Whitecap Books, 1995).

Rita Buchanan, *Better Homes and Gardens Step-By-Step Successful Gardening: Vegetables* (Better Homes & Gardens Books, 1995).

Mary Moody, *100 Plants for Quick Growing Gardens* (Crescent Books, 1995).

John Jeavons, *How to Grow More Vegetables: Fruits, Nuts, Berries, Grains, and Other Crops*, 5th ed. (Ten Speed Press, 1995).

Ann Reilly Dines, *Better Homes and Gardens Four Seasons Gardening: A Month-By-Month Guide to Planning, Planting, and Caring for Your Garden* (Better Homes & Gardens Books, 1994).

Raising and Breeding Indoor Plants

John Evans *The Complete Book of Houseplants: A Practical Guide to Selecting and Caring for Houseplants* (Studio, 1994).

Halina Heitz, *Indoor Plants: Flowering and Foliage Varieties for the Home* (Barrons Educational Series, 1991).

Raising and Breeding Pets and Show Animals

Dan Rice, *The Complete Book of Cat Breeding* (Barrons Educational Series, 1997).

Bil Gutman and Anne Canevari Green, *Becoming Your Pet Bird's Best Friend* (Millbrook Press, 1996).

Matthew M. Vriends and M. Heming-Vriends, *Hand-Feeding and Raising Baby Birds: Breeding, Hand-Feeding, Care, and Management* (Barrons Educational Series, 1996).

John Rose and Sarah Pilliner, *Breeding the Competition Horse*, 2nd ed. (Blackwell Science, 1994).

Dr. Herbert R. Axelrod and Mary E. Sweeney, *The Fascination of Breeding Aquarium Fish* (TFH, 1993).

Chris Mattison, *A-Z of Snake Keeping* (Sterling, 1993).

Robert B. Freeman and Toni C. Freeman, *Breeding and Showing Purebred Dogs: More Adventures on the Road to Westminster* (Betterway, 1992).

Miscellaneous crafts

Michael Bennett, *Discovering and Restoring Antique Furniture: A Practical Illustrated Guide for the Buyer and Restorer of Period Antique Furniture* (Cassell Academic, 1996).

Charla Devereaux and Bernie Hephrun, *The Perfume Kit: Create Your Own Unique Fragrances: A Complete Starter Kit* (MacMillan General Reference, 1996).

Dawn Cusick, *The Button Craft Book* (Lark Books, 1996).

Stephanie Harvey and Peter Williams, *Creative Plasterwork* (Lorenz Books, 1996).

Arlene Hamilton Stewart and Annalee Levine, *The Bead Book* (Andrews & McMeel, 1996).

George Shannon and Pat Torlen, *Stained Glass: Projects & Patterns* (Sterling, 1995).

David Constable, *Candlemaking: Creative Designs and Techniques* (Taylor, 1993).

Jim Rowlands and John Crooks, *Big Book of Kites* (St. Martins Press, 1988).

Edward Fletcher, *Lapidary for Beginners* (Sterling, 1984).

Jere Day, *The Complete Book of Rock Crafting* (Sterling, 1976).

Activity Participation
Folk Art and Craft

Stewart Walton and Sally Walton, *Folk Art: Style & Design* (Sterling, 1996).

Aurelia Gomez, *Crafts of Many Cultures: 30 Authentic Craft Projects from Around the World* (Scholastic, 1996).

Nicholas Barnard, *Living With Folk Art: Ethnic Styles from Around the World* (Bulfinch Press, 1991).

Folk Music

Robert A. Stebbins, *The Barbershop Singer: Inside the Social World of a Musical Hobby* (University of Toronto Press, 1996).

Pete Seeger, *The Incompleat Folksinger* (University of Nebraska Press, 1992).

Larry Sandberg and Dick Weissman, *The Folk Music Sourcebook*, updated ed. (Da Capo Press, 1989).

Folk Dance and Morris Dance

Louise Tythacott, *Dance Traditions Around the World* (Thomson Learning, 1995).

Ted Shawn, *16 Dances in 16 Rhythms* (Princeton Book, 1986).

Cecil J. Sharp, *The Morris Book: With a Description of Dances as Performed by the Morrismen of England* (Charles River Books, 1978).

Square Dance

Margot Gunzenhauser, *The Square Dance and Contra Dance Handbook: Calls, Dance Movements, Music Glossary, Bibliography, Discography and Directories* (McFarland, 1996).

Myrna Martin Schild, *Square Dancing Everyone* (Hunter Textbooks, 1987).

Nature Activities (appreciation)

Hiking, Backpacking, Camping

John Long and Michael Hodgson, *The Dayhiker's Handbook: An All-Terrain, All-Season Guide* (McGraw-Hill, 1996).

Michael Mouland, *The Complete Idiot's Guide to Hiking, Camping, and the Great Outdoors* (Alpha Books, 1996).

Victoria Logue, *Backpacking in the '90s: Tips, Techniques & Secrets*, 3rd ed. (Menasha Ridge Press, 1995).

Stephen Gorman, *Amc Guide to Winter Camping: Wilderness Travel and Adventure in the Cold-Weather Months* (Appalachian Mountain Club, 1991).

Cliff Jacobson, *The Basic Essentials of Map and Compass* (ICS Books, 1988).

Spelunking

Michael R. Taylor, *Cave Passages: Roaming the Underground Wilderness* (Vintage Books, 1997).

National Speleological Society, *Caving Basics*, 3rd ed. (National Speleological Society, 1992).

Bird-Watching

Jan Mahnken, *The Backyard Bird-Lover's Guide* (Storey Communications, 1996).

Sandy Cortright, *Birding Basics* (Sterling, 1995).

Paul Ehrlich, David Dobkin and Darryl Wheye, *The Birder's Handbook: A Field Guide to the Natural History of North American Birds; Including All Species That Regularly Breed North of Mexico* (Fireside, 1988).

Skin (Scuba) Diving and Snorkeling

Dennis K. Graver, *Scuba Diving* (Human Kinetics, 1993).

M. Timothy O'Keefe, *Diving to Adventure!: How to Get the Most Fun from Your Diving & Snorkling* (Larsens Outdoor, 1992).

Snowshoeing

Sally Edwards and Melissa McKenzie, *Snowshoeing* (Human Kinetics, 1995).

Nature Activities (challenges)

Ballooning, Flying and Gliding

Phyllis J. Perry, *Soaring* (Franklin Watts, 1997).

Robert F. Whelan, *Cloud Dancing: Your Introduction to Gliding and Motorless Flight* (Rainbow Books, 1996).

Robert Mark, *The Joy of Flying*, 3rd ed. (Tab Books, 1994)

Christie Costanzo, *Hot Air Ballooning* (Capstone Press, 1989).

Model Airplane Flying

Charles Allison and Andy Nicholls, *Flying Radio Control Aerobatics* (Motorbooks International, 1990).

David Boddington, *Basic Radio Control Flying* (Motorbooks International, 1989).

Surfing

Doug Werner, *Surfer's Start-Up: A Beginner's Guide to Surfing* (Tracks, 1993).

Nick Carroll, *The Next Wave: The World of Surfing* (Abbeville Press, 1991).

Parachuting and Skydiving

Dan Poynter, *Parachuting: The Skydiver's Handbook*, 6th ed. (Para, 1992).

Jim Bates, *Parachuting: From Student to Skydiver* (Tab Books, 1990).

Hang Gliding

Bob Italia, *Hang Gliding* (Abdo & Daughters, 1994).

Toni Will-Harris, *Hang Gliding and Parasailing* (Capstone Press, 1992).

Mountain Climbing

Walt Unsworth, *Hold the Heights: The Foundations of Mountaineering* (Mountaineers Books, 1994).

Don Graydon (ed.), *Mountaineering: The Freedom of the Hills*, 5th ed. (Mountaineers Books, 1992).

Dirt (Trail) Bike Riding (non-competitive)

Jesse Young, *Dirt Bikes* (Capstone Press, 1995).

Nature Activities (exploitation)

Fishing

Ken Schultz, *The Art of Trolling: A Complete Guide to Freshwater* Methods and Tackle, 2nd ed. (McGraw-Hill, 1996).

Tom McNally, *The Complete Book of Fly Fishing*, 2nd ed. (Tab Books, 1993).

Erwin A. Bauer and Bob Stearns, *The Saltwater Fisherman's Bible*, 3rd ed. (Doubleday, 1991).

Cliff Hauptman, *Basic Freshwater Fishing: Step-By-Step Guide to Tackle and Know-How That Catch the Favorite Fish in Your Area* (Stackpole Books, 1988).

Hunting

Dwight R. Schuh (ed.), *Bowhunting Equipment & Skills* (Cowles Creative, 1997).

Edward K. Roggenkamp, III, *American Roughshooting* (Howell Book House, 1996).

Chris Dorsey, *Pheasant Days* (Voyageur Press, 1994).

Al Hofacker (ed.), *Deer & Deer Hunting: A Hunter's Guide to Deer Behavior and Hunting Techniques* (Krause, 1993).

Robert Elman, *The Game Bird Hunter's Bible* (Doubleday, 1993).

Trapping

James A. Bateman, *Trapping: A Practical Guide* (Stackpole Books, 1979).

George Lawson, *Trapping and Tracking* (New Win, 1977).

Mushroom Gathering

Thomas Laessoe, Anna Del Conte and Gary Lincoff, *The Mushroom Book* (Dorling-Kindersley, 1996).

Kent H. McKnight and Vera B. McKnight, *A Field Guide to Mushrooms in North America* (Houghton Mifflin, 1987).

Corporeal Activities

Ice and Roller Skating

Cam Millar and Bruce Curtis, *In-Line Skating Basics* (Sterling, 1996).

Cam Millar and Bruce Curtis, *Roller Hockey* (Sterling, 1996).

Karin Kunzle-Watson and Stephen J. Dearmond, *Ice Skating: Steps to Success* (Human Kinetics, 1995).

Gymnastics, Tumbling and Acrobatics (for gymnastics see Individual Sports – Elite Amateur)

Ivan Bulloch and Diane James, *An Acrobat (I Want to Be)* (World Book, 1995).

Jack Wiley, *Individual Tumbling, Balancing, and Acrobatics* (Solipaz, 1991).

Ballroom Dancing *(see Entertainment – Dance)*

Competitors in Sports, Games and Contests

Polo

Frank Milburn, *Polo: The Emperor of Games* (Knopf, 1994).

Harry Disston, *Beginning Polo* (Oak Tree, 1973).

Curling

Roy E. Thiessen, *Curling Handbook for Curlers, Teachers, and Coaches* (Big Country Books, 1977).

Lacrosse

Jim Hinkson, *Lacrosse Fundamentals* (Warwick, 1993) (dist. by Firefly Books).

Darts

Derek Brown, *Darts* (ICS Books, 1997).

Chris Carey, *The American Darts Organization Book of Darts* (Lyons & Burford, 1993).

Pool/Billiards/Snooker

Steve Mizerak and Joel H. Cohen, *Billiards for Beginners* (ICS Books, 1996).

Robert Byrne, *Byrne's Book of Great Pool Stories* (Harvest Books, 1995).

John Spencer, *Snooker* (NTC, 1993).

Steve Mizerak and Michael E. Panozzo, *Steve Mizerak's Complete Book of Pool* (Contemporary Books, 1990).

Croquet

Steve Boga, *Croquet* (Stackpole Books, 1995).

Donald C. Richardson, *Croquet: The Art and Elegance of Playing the Game* (Harmony Books, 1988).

Handball *(see Individual Sports, elite amateur)*

Race Walking

Scott Roberts, *Fitness Walking* (Masters Press, 1995).

Casey Meyers, *Aerobic Walking: The Best and Safest Weight Loss and Cardiovascular Exercise for Everyone Overweight or Out of Shape* (Vintage Books, 1987).

Long-Distance Running

Lyle J. Micheli and Mark Jenkins, *Healthy Runner's Handbook* (Human Kinetics, 1996).

Bill Rodgers and Scott Douglas, *Bill Rodgers' Lifetime Running Plan: Definitive Programs for Runners of All Ages and Levels* (HarperCollins, 1996).

James F. Fixx, *The Complete Book of Running* (Random House, 1977).

Shooting (see also Individual Sports – Elite Amateur)

The Gun Digest, *The Gun Digest Book of Trap and Skeet Shooting*, 3rd ed. (DBI Books, 1994).

Michael Pearce, *Sporting Clays: Expert Techniques for Every Kind of Clays Course* (Stackpole Books, 1991).

Ping Pong (table tennis)

Gail McCulloch, *Ping Pong* (ICS Books, 1997).

Larry Hodges, *Table Tennis: Steps to Success* (Human Kinetics, 1993).

Orienteering

Tom Renfrew, *Orienteering* (Human Kinetics, 1996).

Bjorn Kjellstrom, *Be Expert With Map & Compass: The Complete Orienteering Handbook*, rev. ed. (MacMillan General Reference, 1994).

Martial Arts (see Individual Sports, elite amateur)

Dog Racing

Elizabeth Ring, *Sled Dogs: Arctic Athletes* (Millbrook Press, 1994).

Thomas A. Walsh, *Greyhound Racing: For Fun and Profit* (Liberty, 1991).

Michael Cooper, *Racing Sled Dogs* (Clarion Books, 1988).

Ice Boating

Natalie Levy, *Iceboating: Your Guide to the Fundamentals and Fine Points of Buying, Sailing, Racing, and Maintaining Your Craft* (David McKay, 1978).

Jack Andresen, *Sailing on Ice* (Oak Tree, 1976).

Power Boat Racing

Jay H. Smith, *Powerboat Racing* (Capstone Press, 1995).

T.J. Andersen, *Power Boat Racing* (Crestwood House, 1988).

Model Racing

David Thomas, *Basics of Radio Control Power Boat Modeling*, 2nd ed. (Kalmbach, 1992).

John Carroll, *Building and Racing Electric Cars and Trucks* (Kalmbach, 1991).

Don Berliner, *Flying Model Airplanes* (Lerner, 1982).

Julie Morgan, *Model Airplane Racing* (Lippincott-Raven, 1972).

Games, Puzzles and Mazes

Card Games

Peter Arnold, *The Book of Card Games* (Hippocrene Books, 1995).

Edmond Hoyle (ed.), Richard L. Frey, Geoffrey Mott-Smith and Albert L. Morehead, *The New Complete Hoyle Revised: The Authoritative Guide to the Official Rules of All Popular Games of Skill and Change*, rev. ed. (Doubleday, 1991).

Oswald Jacoby and James Jacoby, *Jacoby on Card Games* (Pocket Books, 1989).

Backgammon

Bill Robertie, *Backgammon for Winners*, 2nd ed. (Cardoza, 1995).

Chess and Checkers

Laszlo Polgar, *Chess: 5334 Problems, Combinations, and Games* (Black Dog & Leventhal, 1995).

Fred Reinfeld, *Beginners Guide to Winning Chess*, rev. ed. (Foulsham, 1994).

Bill Robertie, *Beginning Chess Play* (Cardoza, 1994).

Vladimir M. Kaplan, *Play Checkers and Win* (Vladimir Kaplan, 1988).

Cribbage

Joseph P. Wergin, *How to Win at Cribbage* (New Win, 1980).

Rummy

Samuel Fry, *Gin Rummy: How to Play and Win* (Dover, 1978).

Solitaire

Douglas Brown, *150 Solitaire Games* (Barnes & Noble, 1992).

Poker and Blackjack

Mike Caro, *Caro's Fundamental Secrets of Winning Poker*, new ed. (Cardoza, 1996).

Henry Tamburin, *Blackjack: Take the Money and Run* (Research Services Unlimited, 1994).

Bridge

Edwin Silberstang, *Handbook of Winning Bridge: A Comprehensive Guide for Beginning and Intermediate Players* (Cardoza, 1995).

Alan Truscott, *Contract Bridge for Beginners and Intermediate Players* (Lifetime Books, 1993).

Scrabble

Joe Edley and John D. Williams, Jr., *Everything Scrabble* (Pocket Books, 1995).

Charades

Michael Johnstone, *Charades and Party Games* (Ward Lock, 1990).

Role-Playing Games

Lawrence Schick, *Heroic Worlds: A History and Guide to Role Playing Games* (Prometheus Books, 1991).

Rick Swan, *The Complete Guide to Role-Playing Games* (St. Martins Press, 1990).

Dominoes

Reiner F. Muller, *Dominoes: Basic Rules & Variations* (Sterling, 1995).

Puzzles, Mazes and Brain Twisters

P. A. Heuser, *3-D Space Mazes* (Dover, 1996).

Stanley Newman (ed.), *Brain Twisters from the World Puzzle Championships*, Vol. 2 (Times Books, 1995).

no author given, *Brain Twisters from the First World Puzzle Championships* (Times Books, 1993).

Will Shortz (ed.) and Rolf Heimann, *Amazing Mazes: Mind Bending Mazes for Ages 6-60* (Troll Associates, 1991).

Dell Books, *The Best of Dell Crossword Puzzles* (Dell Books, 1990).

Linda Hannas, *The Jigsaw Puzzle Book* (Doubleday, 1981).

Liberal Arts Hobbies

Cuisine

Jillian Powell, *Food (Traditions Around the World)* (Thomson Learning, 1995).

Brigid Allen (ed.), *Food: An Oxford Anthology* (Oxford University Press, 1995).

Stephen Mennell, *All Manners of Food: Eating and Taste in England and France from the Middle Ages to the Present*, 2nd ed. (University of Illinois Press, 1995).

Charles Camp, *American Foodways: What, When, Why and How We Eat in America* (August House, 1989).

Beverages – Wine

Gail Bradney (ed.), *Best Wines!: Gold Medal Winners from the Leading Competitions Worldwide* (Print Project, 1996).

Joanna Simon, *Discovering Wine: A Refreshingly Unfussy Beginner's Guide to Finding, Tasting, Judging, Storing, Serving, Cellaring, and, Most of All, Discovering* (Fireside, 1995).

Barbara Ensrud, *Best Wine Buys for $12 and Under: A Guide for the Frugal Connoisseur*, rev. ed. (Villard Books, 1995).

Beverages – Beer

Stuart A. Kallen, *The 50 Greatest Beers in the World: An Expert's Ranking of the Very Best* (Citadel Press, 1996).

Stephen Snyder, *The Beer Companion: A Connoisseur's Guide to the World's Finest Craft Beers* (Siress, 1996).

Peter LaFrance, *Beer Basics: A Quick and Easy Guide* (John Wiley, 1995).

Language

Anatole Lyovin, *An Introduction to the Languages of the World* (Oxford University Press, 1997).

David Crystal, *The Cambridge Encyclopedia of Language*, 2nd ed. (Cambridge University Press, 1997).

Bernard Comrie (ed.), *The Atlas of Languages: The Origin and Development of Languages Throughout the World* (Facts on File, 1996).

Barry Farber, *How to Learn Any Language: Quickly, Easily, Inexpensively, Enjoyably and on Your Own* (Citadel Press, 1991).

Science

R.C. Olby, G.N. Cantor and J.R.R. Christie (eds.), *Companion to the History of Modern Science* (Routledge, 1996).

John Horgan, *The End of Science: Facing the Limits of Knowledge in the Twilight of the Scientific Age* (Addison-Wesley, 1996).

John Kelly and Steve Parker, *Shocking Science: 5,000 Years of Mishaps and Misunderstandings* (Turner, 1996).

Anthony M. Alioto, *A History of Western Science*, 2nd ed. (Prentice Hall, 1992).

Philosophy

Albert B. Hakim, *Historical Introduction to Philosophy*, 3rd ed. (Prentice Hall, 1996).

James A. Gould (ed.), *Classic Philosophical Questions*, 8th ed. (Prentice Hall, 1995).

Bryan Magee, *The Great Philosophers: An Introduction to Western Philosophy* (Oxford University Press, 1988).

Literature

Andrew Bennett and Nicholas Royle, *An Introduction to Literature, Criticism, and Theory: Key Critical Concepts* (Prentice Hall, 1996).

William Harmon, C. Hugh Holman, William Flint Thrall and Addi

Hibbard, *A Handbook to Literature*, 7th ed. (Prentice Hall, 1995).

Sue Collins, *Approaching Literature* (Teach Yourself Books, 1993).

Kenneth Rexroth, *Classics Revisited* (New Directions, 1986).

Politics

Richard J. Ellis, *American Political Cultures* (Oxford University Press, 1996).

Stephen Hess and Sandy Northrop, *Drawn & Quartered: The History of American Political Cartoons* (Elliott & Clark, 1996).

James L. Sundquist, *Dynamics of the Party System: Alignment and Realignment of Political Parties in the United States*, rev. ed. (Brookings Institute, 1983).

Career Volunteering

Robert Wuthnow, *Learning to Care: Elementary Kindness in an Age of Indifference* (Oxford University Press, 1995).

Jeffrey Hollender and Linda Catling, *How to Make the World a Better Place: 116 Ways You Can Make a Difference* (W.W. Norton, 1995).

Steve Fiffer and Sharon S. Fiffer, *50 Ways to Help Your Community: A Handbook for Change* (Doubleday, 1994).

Andrew Carroll, *Golden Opportunities: A Volunteer Guide for Americans over 50* (Petersons Guides, 1994).

Milton Meltzer, *Who Cares? Millions Do . . . A Book about Altruism* (Walker, 1994).

Darcy C. Devney, *The Volunteer's Survival Manual: The Only Practical Guide to Giving Your Time and Money* (Practical Press, 1992).

Joan Wolfe, *Making Things Happen: How to Be an Effective Volunteer* (Island Press, 1991).

John Raynolds, III and Eleanor Raynolds, *Beyond Success: How Volunteer Service Can Help You Begin Making a Life Instead of a Living* (Master Media, 1988).

Works Cited

Aronowitz, Stanley, and William DiFazio. 1994. *The Jobless Future: Sci-Tech and the Dogma of Work*. Minneapolis: University of Minnesota Press.

Bellah, Robert N., Richard Madsen, William A. Sullivan, Ann Swidler and Steven M. Tipton. 1985. *Habits of the Heart: Individualism and Commitment in American Life*. Berkeley: University of California Press.

Brightbill, Charles K. 1961. *Man and Leisure: A Philosophy of Recreation*. Englewood Cliffs, NJ: Prentice-Hall (pp.v-vi).

Calgary Herald. 1988. "Volunteers Armed by Worried Police." 25 February, A2.

Carp, F.M. 1968. "Differences among Older Workers, Volunteers, and Persons Who are Neither." *Journal of Gerontology* 23: 497-501.

Carrier, Roch. 1995. "What Price Culture?" *The Financial Post* (28 October): 23.

Csikszentmihalyi, Mihaly. 1975. *Beyond Boredom and Anxiety: The Experience of Play in Work and Games*. San Francisco: Jossey-Bass.

Dannefer, Dale. 1980. "Rationality and Passion in Private Experience: Modern Consciousness and the Social World of Old-Car Collectors." *Social Problems* 27: 392-412.

Deegan, Mary Jo, and Larry E. Nutt. 1975. "The Hospital Volunteer." *Sociology of Work and Occupations* 2: 338-353.

Dubin, Robert. 1992. *Central Life Interests: Creative Individualism in a Complex World*. New Brunswick, NJ: Transaction Publishers (pp. 41-42).

Elgin, Duane. 1981. *Voluntary Simplicity: Toward a Way of Life That is Outwardly Simple, Inwardly Rich*. New York: William Morrow.

Fine, Gary A. 1983. *Shared Fantasy: Role-Playing Games as Social Worlds*. Chicago: University of Chicago Press.

——. 1988. "Dying for a Laugh." *Western Folklore* 47: 177-194.

Finnegan, Ruth. 1989. *The Hidden Musicians: Music-Making in an English Town*. Cambridge: Cambridge University Press.

Floro, George K. 1978. "What to look for in a Study of the Volunteer in the Work World." Pp. 194-202 in *The Small City and Regional Community*, ed. R.P. Wolensky and E.J. Miller. Stevens Point, WI: Foundation Press.

Fodor Travel Publications. 1994. *Fodor's Great American Learning Vacations*. New York: Fodor Travel Publications.

Forster, E.M. 1961. *A Passage to India*. Harmondsworth, Eng.: Penguin.

Glasser, Ralph. 1970. *Leisure: Penalty or Prize?* London: Macmillan.

Glyptis, Sue. 1989. *Leisure and Unemployment*. Milton Keynes, Eng.: Open University Press.

Godbout, Jacques. 1986. "La Participation: Instrument de Professionalisation des Loisirs." *Loisir et Société/Society and Leisure* 9: 33-40.

Goffman, Erving. 1963. *Stigma: Notes on the Management of Spoiled Identity*. Englewood Cliffs, NJ: Prentice-Hall.

Gordon, Charles. 1992. "Another Major Step Forward: Taking the Fun out of Leisure." *Ottawa Citizen* (Sunday, 21 June): 19.

Hamilton-Smith, Elery. 1971. "The Preparation of Volunteer Workers with Adolescent Groups." *Australian Social Work* 24 (3-4): 26-33.

Haworth, John T. 1986. "Meaningful Activity and Psychological Models of Non-Employed." *Leisure Studies* 5: 281-297.

Hinton-Braaten, Kathleen. 1980. "Symphony Auditions: A Tough Way to Go." *International Musician* 79 (July): 5.

Holtz, Janicemarie A. 1975. "The 'Professional' Duplicate Bridge Player." *Urban Life* 4: 131-148.

Howard, Ann (ed.). 1995. *The Changing Nature of Work*. San Francisco: Jossey-Bass.

Howe, Christine. 1995. "Factors Impacting Leisure in Middle Aged Adults throughout the World: United States." *World Leisure & Recreation* 37 (1): 37-38.

Huizinger, Johan. 1955. *Homo Ludens: A Study of the Play Element in Culture*. Boston: Beacon.

Jenkins, Clive, and Barry Sherman. 1979. *The Collapse of Work*. London: Eyre Methuen.

———. 1981. *The Leisure Shock*. London: Eyre Methuen.

Jones, Barry. 1982. *Sleepers Wake! Technology and the Future of Work*. Melbourne, Aus.: Oxford University Press.

Kay, Tess. 1990. "Active Unemployment – A Leisure Pattern for the Future." *Loisir et Société / Society and Leisure* 12: 413-30.

Kouri, Mary K. 1990. *Volunteerism and Older Adults*. Santa Barbara, CA: ABC-CLIO.

Lalive D'Epinay, Christian J. 1992. "Beyond the Antinomy: Work versus Leisure?" *Loisir et Société / Society and Leisure* 14: 433-446.

Lankford, John. 1979. "Amateur Versus Professional: The Transatlantic Debate over the Measure of Jovian Longitude." *Journal of the British Astronomical Association* 89: 574-582.

Lauffer, Armand, and Sarah Gorodezky. 1990. *Volunteers*. Beverly Hills, CA: Sage.

Lefkowitz, Bernard. 1979. *Breaktime*. New York: Penguin.

Levine, Shar, and Leslie Johnstone. 1995. *Silly Science: Strange and Startling Projects to Amaze Your Family and Friends*. New York: Wiley.

Machlowitz, Marilyn. 1980. *Workaholics: Living with Them, Working with Them*. Reading, MA: Addison-Wesley.

Mahoney, Michael. 1976. *Scientist as Subject: The Psychological Imperative*. Cambridge, MA: Ballinger.

Marsh, Leonard. 1972. *At Home with Music*. Vancouver: Versatile Publishing Co.

Menzies, Hugh D. 1996. "Who'll Plug the Safety-Net Hole?" *Financial Post* (November 23): 30.

Mittelstaedt, Robin D. 1995. "Reenacting the American Civil War: A Unique Form of Serious Leisure for Adults." *World Leisure & Recreation* 37 (1): 23-27.

Moore, Maureen. 1989. "Dual-Earner Families: The New Norm." *Canadian Social Trends* no. 12 (Spring): 24-26.

Munro, Thomas. 1957. "Four Hundred Arts and Types of Art." *Journal of Aesthetics and Art Criticism* 16:44-65.

Neulinger, John. 1981. *To Leisure: An Introduction*. Boston: Allyn and Bacon (pp. 188-191).

O'Hara, Bruce. 1993. *Working Harder isn't Working!: How We can Save the Environment, the Economy, and Our Sanity by Working Less and Enjoying Life More*. Vancouver, BC: New Star Books.

Olmsted, Allan D. 1988. "Morally Controversial Leisure: The Social World of Gun Collectors." *Symbolic Interaction* 11: 277-288.

———. 1991. "Collecting: Leisure, Investment, or Obsession?" *Journal of Social Behavior and Personality* 6: 287-306.

Overs, Robert P. 1984. *Guide to Avocational Activities*. Sussex, WI: Signpost Press

Pearce, Jone. 1993. *Volunteers: The Organizational Behavior of Unpaid Workers*. London and New York: Routledge.

Reid, Donald G., and Roger C. Mannell. 1994. "The Globalization of the Economy and Potential New Roles for Work and Leisure." *Loisir et Société / Society and Leisure*, 17: 251-268.

Richards, Roy. 1993. *101 Science Surprises: Exciting Experiments with Everyday Materials*. New York: Sterling Publishing Co.

Rifkin, Jeremy. 1995. *The End of Work*. New York: G.P. Putnam's Sons.

Roadburg, Alan. 1985. *Aging: Retirement, Leisure, and Work in Canada*. Toronto: Methuen.

Rosenthal, S.F. 1981. "Marginal or Mainstream: Two Studies of Contemporary Chiropractic." *Sociological Focus* 14: 271-85.

Rothenberg, Marc. 1981. "Organization and Control: Professionals and Amateurs in American Astronomy." *Social Studies in Science* 11: 305-325

Rybczynski, Witold. 1991. *Waiting for the Weekend*. New York: Viking.

Samuel, Nicole. 1994. "The Future of Leisure Time." Pp. 45-57 in *New Routes for Leisure*. Lisbon, Portugal: Instituto de Ciências Sociais da Universidade de Lisboa.

Sarlo, Christopher. 1992. *Poverty in Canada*. Vancouver, BC: Fraser Institute.

Schor, Juliet B. 1991. *The Overworked American: The Unexpected Decline of Leisure*. New York: Basic Books.

Shamir, Boas. 1985. "Unemployment and 'free time' – The Role of the Protestant Ethic and Work Involvement." *Leisure Studies* 4: 333-345.

Sheehy, Gail. 1995. *New Passages: Mapping Your Life Across Time*. New York: Random House.

Sherman, Barry. 1986. *Working at Leisure*. London: Methuen London Ltd.

Sobel, Michael E. 1981. *Lifestyle and Social Structure: Concepts, Definitions, Analyses*. New York: Academic Press.

Statistics Canada. 1980. *An Overview of Volunteer Workers in Canada*, cat. no. 71-530. Ottawa: Minister of Supply and Services.

Stebbins, Robert A. 1978. "Classical Music Amateurs: A Definitional Study." *Humboldt Journal of Social Relations* 5: 78-103.

——-. 1978. "Creating High Culture: The American Amateur Classical Musician." *Journal of American Culture* 1: 616-631.

——-. 1979. *Amateurs: On the Margin Between Work and Leisure*. Beverly Hills, CA: Sage Publications.

——-. 1981. "Toward a Social Psychology of Stage Fright." Pp. 156-163 in *Sport in the Sociocultural Process*, ed. M. Hart and S. Birrell. Dubuque, IO: W.C. Brown.

——-. 1981. "Looking Downwards: Sociological Images of the Vocation and Avocation of Astronomy." *Journal of Royal Astronomical Society of Canada* 75 (February): 2-14.

——-. 1990. *The Laugh-Makers: Stand-Up Comedy as Art, Business, and Life-Style*. Montreal and Kingston: McGill-Queen's University Press.

——-. 1992. *Amateurs, Professionals, and Serious Leisure*. Montreal and Kingston: McGill-Queen's University Press.

——-. 1993. *Career, Culture and Social Psychology in a Variety Art: The Magician*. Malabar, FL: Krieger Publishing Co.

——-. 1993. *Canadian Football: The View from the Helmet*. Toronto: Canadian Scholars' Press.

——-. 1994. "The Liberal Arts Hobbies: A Neglected Subtype of Serious Leisure." *Loisir et Société/Society and Leisure* 16: 173-186.

——-. 1994. *The Franco-Calgarians: French Language, Leisure, and Linguistic Life-Style in an Anglophone City*. Toronto: University of Toronto Press.

——. 1996. *The Barbershop Singer: Inside the Social World of a Musical Hobby*. Toronto: University of Toronto Press.

——. 1996. *Tolerable Differences: Living with Deviance*, 2nd ed. Toronto, ON: McGraw-Hill Ryerson.

——. 1996. "Cultural Tourism as Serious Leisure." *Annals of Tourism Research* 23: 948-950

——. 1996. "Volunteering: A Serious Leisure Perspective." *Nonprofit and Voluntary Sector Quarterly* 25: 211-224.

——. 1997. "Casual Leisure: A Conceptual Statement." *Leisure Studies* 16: 17-25.

——. 1997. "Lifestyle as a Generic Concept in Ethnographic Research." *Quality and Quantity* 31: 347-360.

Thompson, Shona. 1992. "'Mum's Tennis Day': The Gendered Definition of Older Women's Leisure." *Loisir et Société / Society and Leisure* 15: 271-289.

Unruh, David R. 1979. "Characteristics and Types of Participation in Social Worlds." *Symbolic Interaction* 2: 115-130.

——. 1980. "The Nature of Social Worlds." *Pacific Sociological Review* 23: 271-296.

U.S. Bureau of the Census. 1995. *Statistical Abstract of the United States: 1995*, 115th ed. Washington, D.C.

U.S. National Institute of Law Enforcement and Criminal Justice. 1977. *Citizen Patrol Projects: National Evaluation Program*. Washington, D.C.: U.S. Government Printing Office.

Van Til, Jon. 1988. *Mapping the Third Sector: Voluntarism in a Changing Political Economy*. New York: The Foundation Center.

Veal, A.J. 1993. The Concept of Lifestyle: A Review. *Leisure Studies* 12: 233-252.

Walpole, Brenda. 1988. *175 Science Experiments to Amuse and Amaze Your Friends: Experiments, Tricks, Things to Make*. New York: Random House.

Williams, Joyce L. 1987. "An Uneasy Balance: Voluntarism and and Professionalism." *American Archivist* 50 (Winter): 7-10.

Williams, Thomas R. 1983. "Astronomers as Amateurs." *The Journal of the American Association of Variable Star Observers* 12: 1-4.

Yankelovich, Daniel. 1981. *New Rules: Searching for Self-Fulfillment in a World Turned Upside Down.* New York: Random House.

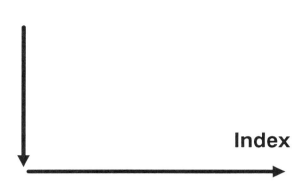

Index